£29

RB
145
THE

...ucation and Training
...rary

Withdrawn

D1339323

T03624

Thieme

Color Atlas of Hematology

Practical Microscopic and Clinical Diagnosis

Harald Theml, M.D.
Professor, Private Practice
Hematology/Oncology
Munich, Germany

Heinz Diem, M.D.
Klinikum Grosshadern
Institute of Clinical Chemistry
Munich, Germany

Torsten Haferlach, M.D.
Professor, Klinikum Grosshadern
Laboratory for Leukemia Diagnostics
Munich, Germany

2nd revised edition

262 color illustrations
32 tables

Thieme
Stuttgart · New York

Library of Congress Cataloging-in-Publication Data is available from the publisher

This book is an authorized revised translation of the 5th German edition published and copyrighted 2002 by Thieme Verlag, Stuttgart, Germany.
Title of the German edition:
Taschenatlas der Hämatologie

Translator: Ursula Peter-Czichi PhD, Atlanta, GA, USA

1st German edition 1983
2nd German edition 1986
3rd German edition 1991
4th German edition 1998
5th German edition 2002
1st English edition 1985
1st French edition 1985
2nd French edition 2000
1st Indonesion edition 1989
1st Italian edition 1984
1st Japanese edition 1997

© 2004 Georg Thieme Verlag
Rüdigerstraße 14, 70469 Stuttgart,
Germany
http://www.thieme.de

Thieme New York, 333 Seventh Avenue,
New York, NY 10001 USA
http://www.thieme.com

Cover design: Cyclus, Stuttgart
Typesetting and printing in Germany by
Druckhaus Götz GmbH, Ludwigsburg

ISBN 3-13-673102-6 (GTV)
ISBN 1-58890-193-9 (TNY)   1 2 3 4 5

Important note: Medicine is an ever-changing science undergoing continual development. Research and clinical experience are continually expanding our knowledge, in particular our knowledge of proper treatment and drug therapy. Insofar as this book mentions any dosage or application, readers may rest assured that the authors, editors, and publishers have made every effort to ensure that such references are in accordance with **the state of knowledge at the time of production of the book.**

Nevertheless, this does not involve, imply, or express any guarantee or responsibility on the part of the publishers in respect to any dosage instructions and forms of applications stated in the book. **Every user is requested to examine carefully** the manufacturers' leaflets accompanying each drug and to check, if necessary in consultation with a physician or specialist, whether the dosage schedules mentioned therein or the contraindications stated by the manufacturers differ from the statements made in the present book. Such examination is particularly important with drugs that are either rarely used or have been newly released on the market. Every dosage schedule or every form of application used is entirely at the user's own risk and responsibility. The authors and publishers request every user to report to the publishers any discrepancies or inaccuracies noticed.

Some of the product names, patents, and registered designs referred to in this book are in fact registered trademarks or proprietary names even though specific reference to this fact is not always made in the text. Therefore, the appearance of a name without designation as proprietary is not to be construed as a representation by the publisher that it is in the public domain.

This book, including all parts thereof, is legally protected by copyright. Any use, exploitation, or commercialization outside the narrow limits set by copyright legislation, without the publisher's consent, is illegal and liable to prosecution. This applies in particular to photostat reproduction, copying, mimeographing, preparation of microfilms, and electronic data processing and storage.

Preface

Our Current Edition

Although this is the second English edition of our hematology atlas, this edition is *completely new*. As an immediate sign of this change, there are now three authors. The completely updated visual presentation uses digital images, and the content is organized according to the most up-to-date morphological classification criteria.

In this new edition, our newly formed team of authors from Munich (the "Munich Group") has successfully shared their knowledge with you. Heinz Diem and Torsten Haferlach are nationally recognized as lecturers of the diagnostics curriculum of the German Association for Hematology and Oncology.

Goals

Most physicians are fundamentally "visually oriented." Apart from immediate patient care, the microscopic analysis of blood plays to this preference. This explains the delight and level of involvement on the part of practitioners in the pursuit of morphological analyses.

Specialization notwithstanding, the hematologist wants to preserve the opportunity to perform groundbreaking diagnostics in hematology for the general practitioner, surgeon, pediatrician, the MTA technician, and all medical support personnel. New colleagues must also be won to the cause. Utmost attention to the analysis of hematological changes is essential for a timely diagnosis.

Even before bone marrow cytology, cytochemistry, or immunocytochemistry, information based on the analysis of blood is of immediate relevance in the doctor's office. It is central to the diagnosis of the diseases of the blood cell systems themselves, which make their presence known through changes in blood components.

The exhaustive quantitative and qualitative use of hematological diagnostics is crucial. Discussions with colleagues from all specialties and teaching experience with advanced medical students confirm its importance. In cases where a diagnosis remains elusive, the awareness of the next diagnostic step becomes relevant. Then, further investigation through bone marrow, lymph node, or organ tissue cytology can yield firm results. This pocket atlas offers the basic knowledge for the use of these techniques as well.

Organization

Reflecting our goals, the inductive organization proceeds from simple to specialized diagnostics. By design, we subordinated the description of the bone marrow cytology to the diagnostic blood analysis (CBC). However, we have responded to feedback from readers of the previous editions and have included the principles of bone marrow diagnostics and non-ambiguous clinical bone marrow findings so that frequent and relevant diagnoses can be quickly made, understood, or replicated.

The nosology and differential diagnosis of hematological diseases are presented to you in a tabular form. We wanted to offer you a pocketbook for everyday work, not a reference book. Therefore, morphological curiosities, or anomalies, are absent in favor of a practical approach to morphology. The cellular components of organ biopsies and exudates are briefly discussed, mostly as a reminder of the importance of these tests.

The images are consistently photographed as they normally appear in microscopy (magnification 100 or 63 with oil immersion lens, occasionally master-detail magnification objective 10 or 20). Even though surprising perspectives sometimes result from viewing cells at a higher magnification, the downside is that this by no means facilitates the recognition of cells using your own microscope.

Instructions for the Use of this Atlas

The organization of this atlas supports a systematic approach to the study of hematology (see Table of Contents). The index offers ways to answer detailed questions and access the hematological terminology with references to the main description and further citations.

The best way to become familiar with your pocket atlas is to first have a cursory look through its entire content. The images are accompanied by short legends. On the pages opposite the images you will find corresponding short descriptive texts and tables. This text portion describes cell phenomena and discusses in more detail further diagnostic steps as well as the diagnostic approach to disease manifestations.

Acknowledgments

Twenty years ago, Professor Herbert Begemann dedicated the foreword to the first edition of this hematology atlas. He acknowledged that—beyond cell morphology—this atlas aims at the clinical picture of patients. We are grateful for being able to continue this tradition, and for the impulses from our teachers and companions that make this possible.

We thank our colleagues: J. Rastetter, W. Kaboth, K. Lennert, H. Löffler, H. Heimpel, P.M. Reisert, H. Brücher, W. Enne, T. Binder, H.D. Schick, W. Hiddemann, D. Seidel.

Munich, January 2004   Harald Theml, Heinz Diem, Torsten Haferlach

Contents

Physiology and Pathophysiology of Blood Cells: Methods and Test Procedures

Introduction to the Physiology and Pathophysiology of the Hematopoietic System

The reason why quantitative and qualitative diagnosis based on the cellular components of the blood is so important is that blood cells are easily accessible indicators of disturbances in their organs of origin or degradation—which are much less easily accessible. Thus, disturbances in the erythrocyte, granulocyte, and thrombocyte series allow important conclusions to be drawn about bone marrow function, just as disturbances of the lymphatic cells indicate reactions or disease states of the specialized lymphopoietic organs (basically, the lymph nodes, spleen, and the diffuse lymphatic intestinal organ).

Cell Systems

All blood cells derive from a common stem cell. Under the influences of local and humoral factors, stem cells differentiate into different

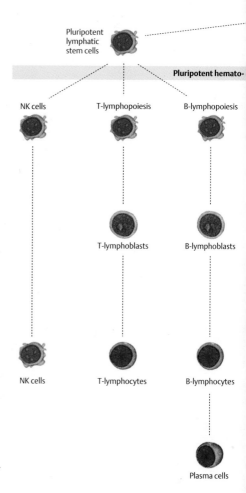

Fig. **1** Model of cell lineages ▶ in hematopoiesis

cell lines (Fig. **1**). Erythropoiesis and thrombopoiesis proceed independently once the stem cell stage has been passed, whereas monocytopoiesis and granulocytopoiesis are quite closely "related." Lymphocytopoiesis is the most independent among the remaining cell series. Granulocytes, monocytes, and lymphocytes are collectively called leukocytes (white blood cells), a term that has been retained since the days before staining

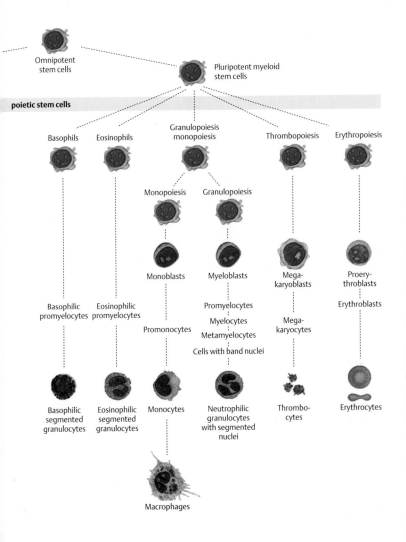

Omnipotent stem cells

Pluripotent myeloid stem cells

poietic stem cells

Basophils   Eosinophils

Granulopoiesis monopoiesis

Thrombopoiesis   Erythropoiesis

Monopoiesis   Granulopoiesis

Monoblasts   Myeloblasts   Mega-karyoblasts   Proery-throblasts

Basophilic promyelocytes   Eosinophilic promyelocytes

Promyelocytes
Myelocytes
Metamyelocytes
Cells with band nuclei

Promonocytes

Mega-karyocytes

Erythroblasts

Basophilic segmented granulocytes   Eosinophilic segmented granulocytes   Monocytes   Neutrophilic granulocytes with segmented nuclei   Thrombo-cytes   Erythrocytes

Macrophages

methods were available, when the only distinction that could be made was between erythrocytes (red blood cells) and the rest.

All these cells are eukaryotic, that is, they are made up of a nucleus, sometimes with visible nucleoli, surrounded by cytoplasm, which may include various kinds of organelles, granulations, and vacuoles.

Despite the common origin of all the cells, ordinary light microscopy reveals fundamental and characteristic differences in the nuclear chromatin structure in the different cell series and their various stages of maturation (Fig. 2).

The developing cells in the granulocyte series (myeloblasts and promyelocytes), for example, show a delicate, fine "net-like" (reticular) structure. Careful microscopic examination (using fine focus adjustment to view different depth levels) reveals a detailed nuclear structure that resembles fine or coarse gravel (Fig. 2a). With progressive stages of nuclear maturation in this series (myelocytes, metamyelocytes, and band or staff cells), the chromatin condenses into bands or streaks, giving the nucleus—which at the same time is adopting a characteristic curved shape—a spotted and striped pattern (Fig. 2b).

Lymphocytes, on the other hand—particularly in their circulating forms—always have large, solid-looking nuclei. Like cross-sections through geological slate, homogeneous, dense chromatin bands alternate with lighter interruptions and fissures (Fig. 2c).

Each of these cell series contains precursors that can divide (blast precursors) and mature or almost mature forms that can no longer divide; the morphological differences between these correspond not to steps in mito-

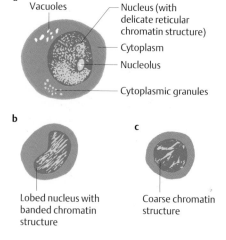

a Vacuoles — Nucleus (with delicate reticular chromatin structure)
— Cytoplasm
— Nucleolus
— Cytoplasmic granules

b Lobed nucleus with banded chromatin structure

c Coarse chromatin structure

Fig. **2**   Principles of cell structure with examples of different nuclear chromatin structure. **a** Cell of the myeloblast to promyelocyte type. **b** Cell of the myelocyte to staff or band cell type. **c** Cell of the lymphocyte type with coarsely structured chromatin

sis, but result from continuous "maturation processes" of the cell nucleus and cytoplasm. Once this is understood, it becomes easier not to be too rigid about morphological distinctions between certain cell stages. The blastic precursors usually reside in the hematopoietic organs (bone marrow and lymph nodes). Since, however, a strict blood–bone marrow barrier does not exist (blasts are kept out of the bloodstream essentially only by their limited plasticity, i.e., their inability to cross the diffusion barrier into the bloodstream), it is in principle possible for any cell type to be found in peripheral blood, and when cell production is increased, the statistical frequency with which they cross into the bloodstream will naturally rise as well. Conventionally, cells are sorted left to right from immature to mature, so an increased level of immature cells in the bloodstream causes a "left shift" in the composition of a cell series—although it must be said that only in the precursor stages of granulopoiesis are the cell morphologies sufficiently distinct for this left shift to show up clearly.

The distribution of white blood cells outside their places of origin cannot be inferred simply from a drop of capillary blood. This is because the majority of white cells remain out of circulation, "marginated" in the epithelial lining of vessel walls or in extravascular spaces, from where they may be quickly recruited back to the bloodstream. This phenomenon explains why white cell counts can vary rapidly without or before any change has taken place in the rate of their production.

Cell functions. A brief indication of the functions of the various cell groups follows (see Table **1**).

Neutrophil granulocytes with segmented nuclei serve mostly *to defend against bacteria*. Predominantly outside the vascular system, in "inflamed" tissue, they phagocytose and lyse bacteria. The blood merely transports the granulocytes to their site of action.

The function of **eosinophilic granulocytes** is *defense against parasites*; they have a direct cytotoxic action on parasites and their eggs and larvae. They also play a role in the *down-regulation of anaphylactic shock reactions* and autoimmune responses, thus controlling the influence of basophilic cells.

The main function of **basophilic granulocytes** and their tissue-bound equivalents (tissue mast cells) is to regulate circulation through the release of substances such as histamine, serotonin, and heparin. These tissue hormones *increase vascular permeability* at the site of various local antigen activity and thus regulate the influx of the other inflammatory cells.

The main function of **monocytes** is the defense against *bacteria, fungi, viruses,* and *foreign bodies*. Defensive activities take place mostly outside the vessels by phagocytosis. Monocytes also break down endogenous cells (e.g., erythrocytes) at the end of their life cycles, and they are assumed to perform a similar function in defense against tumors. Outside the bloodstream, monocytes develop into histiocytes; macrophages in the endothelium of the body cavities; epithelioid cells; foreign body macrophages (including Langhans' giant cells); and many other cells.

Lymphocytes are divided into two major basic groups according to function.

Thymus-dependent T-lymphocytes, which make up about 70% of lymphocytes, provide *local defense against antigens* from organic and inorganic foreign bodies in the form of delayed-type hypersensitivity, as classically exemplified by the tuberculin reaction. T-lymphocytes are divided into helper cells and suppressor cells. The small group of NK (natural killer) cells, which have a direct cytotoxic function, is closely related to the T-cell group.

The other group is the bone-marrow-dependent B-lymphocytes or B-cells, which make up about 20% of lymphocytes. Through their development into immunoglobulin-secreting plasma cells, B-lymphocytes are responsible for the entire *humoral side of defense* against viruses, bacteria, and allergens.

Table **1**   Cells in a normal peripheral blood smear and their physiological roles

Cell type	Function	Count (% of leukocytes)
Neutrophilic band granulocytes (band neutrophil)	Precursors of segmented cells that provide antibacterial immune response	0–4%
Neutrophilic segmented granulocyte (segmented neutrophil)	Phagocytosis of bacteria; migrate into tissue for this purpose	50–70%
Lymphocytes (B- and T-lymphocytes, morphologically indistinguishable)	B-lymphocytes (20% of lymphocytes) mature and form plasma cells → antibody production. T-lymphocytes (70%): cytotoxic defense against viruses, foreign antigens, and tumors.	20–50%
Monocytes	Phagocytosis of bacteria, protozoa, fungi, foreign bodies. Transformation in target tissue	2–8%
Eosinophilic granulocytes	Immune defense against parasites, immune regulation	1–4%
Basophilic granulocytes	Regulation of the response to local inflammatory processes	0–1%

Erythrocytes are the oxygen carriers for all oxygen-dependent metabolic reactions in the organism. They are the only blood cells without nuclei, since this allows them to bind and exchange the greatest number of O_2 molecules. Their physiological biconcave disk shape with a thick rim provides optimal plasticity.

Thrombocytes form the aggregates that, along with humoral coagulation factors, close up vascular lesions. During the aggregation process, in addition to the mechanical function, thrombocytic granules also release factors that promote coagulation.

Thrombocytes develop from polyploid megakaryocytes in the bone marrow. They are the enucleated, fragmented cytoplasmic portions of these progenitor cells.

Principles of Regulation and Dysregulation in the Blood Cell Series and their Diagnostic Implications

Quantitative and qualitative equilibrium between all blood cells is maintained under normal conditions through regulation by humoral factors, which ensure a balance between cell production (mostly in the bone marrow) and cell degradation (mostly in the spleen, liver, bone marrow, and the diffuse reticular tissue).

Compensatory increases in cell production are induced by cell loss or increased cell demand. This compensatory process can lead to qualitative changes in the composition of the blood, e.g., the occurrence of nucleated red cell precursors compensating for blood loss or increased oxygen requirement, or following deficiency of certain metabolites (in the restitution phase, e.g., during iron or vitamin supplementation). Similarly, during acute immune reactions, which lead to an increased demand for cells, immature leukocyte forms may appear ("left shift").

Increased cell counts in one series can lead to *suppression* of cell production in *another series*. The classic example is the suppression of erythrocyte production (the pathomechanical details of which are incompletely understood) during infectious/toxic reactions, which affect the white cells ("infectious anemia").

Metabolite deficiency as a pathogenic stimulus affects the *erythrocyte series* first and most frequently. Although other cell series are also affected, this series, with its high turnover, is the one most vulnerable to metabolite deficiencies. Iron deficiency, for example, rapidly leads to reduced hemoglobin in the erythrocytes, while vitamin B_{12} and/or folic acid deficiency will result in complex disturbances in cell formation. Eventually, these disturbances will start to show effects in the other cell series as well.

Toxic influences on cell production usually affect *all cell series*. The effects of toxic chemicals (including alcohol), irradiation, chronic infections, or tumor load, for example, usually lead to a greater or lesser degree of suppression in all the blood cell series, lymphocytes and thrombocytes being the most resistant. The most extreme result of toxic effects is panmyelophthisis (the synonym "aplastic anemia" ignores the fact that the leukocyte and thrombocyte series are usually also affected).

Autoimmune and allergic processes may *selectively affect* a *single cell series*. Results of this include "allergic" agranulocytosis, immunohemolytic anemia, and thrombocytopenia triggered by either infection or medication. Autoimmune suppression of the pluripotent stem cells can also occur, causing panmyelophthisis.

Malignant dedifferentiation can basically occur in *cells of any lineage at any stage where the cells are able to divide*, causing chronic or acute clinical manifestations. These deviations from normal differentiation occur most frequently in the white cell series, causing "leukemias." Recent data indicate that in fact in these cases the remaining cell series also become distorted, perhaps via generalized atypical stem cell formation. Erythroblastosis, polycythemia, and essential thrombocythemia are examples showing that malignant processes can also manifest themselves primarily in the erythrocyte or thrombocyte series.

Malignant "transformations" always affect blood cell precursors that are still capable of dividing, and the result is an accumulation of identical, constantly self-reproducing blastocytes. These are not necessarily always observed in the bloodstream, but can remain in the bone marrow. That is why, in "leukemia," it is often not the number of cells, but the increasing lack of normal cells that is the indicative hematological finding.

All disturbances of bone marrow function are accompanied by quantitative and/or qualitative changes in the composition of *blood cells* or *blood proteins*. Consequently, in most disorders, careful analysis of changes in the blood together with clinical findings and other laboratory data produces the same information as bone marrow cytology. The relationship between the production site (bone marrow) and the destination (the blood) is rarely so fundamentally disturbed that hematological analysis and humoral parameters will not suffice for a diagnosis. This is virtually always true for *hypoplastic–anaplastic* processes in one or all cell series with resulting cytopenia but without hematological signs of malignant cell proliferation.

Procedures, Assays, and Normal Values

Taking Blood Samples

> Since cell counts are affected by the state of the blood circulation, the conditions under which samples are taken should be the same so far as possible if comparable values are desired.

This means that blood should always be drawn at about the same time of day and after at least eight hours of fasting, since both circadian rhythm and nutritional status can affect the findings. If strictly comparable values are required, there should also be half an hour of bed rest before the sample is drawn, but this is only practicable in a hospital setting. In other settings (i.e., outpatient clinics), bringing portable instruments to the relaxed, seated patient works well.

A sample of capillary blood may be taken when there are no further tests that would require venous access for a larger sample volume. A well-perfused fingertip or an earlobe is ideal; in newborns or young infants, the heel is also a good site. If the circulation is poor, the blood flow can be increased by warming the extremity by immersing it in warm water. Without pressure, the puncture area is swabbed several times with 70% alcohol, and the skin is then punctured firmly but gently with a sterile disposable lancet. The first droplet of blood is discarded because it may be contaminated, and the ensuing blood is drawn into the pipette (see below). Care should be taken not to exert pressure on the tissue from which the blood is being drawn, because this too can change the cell composition of the sample.

Obviously, if a venous blood sample is to be taken for the purposes of other tests, or if an intravenous injection is going to be performed, the blood sample for hematological analysis can be taken from the same site. To do this, the blood is allowed to flow via an intravenous needle into a specially prepared (commercially available) EDTA-treated tube. The tube is filled to the 1-ml mark and then carefully shaken several times. The very small amount of EDTA in the tube prevents the blood from clotting, but can itself be safely ignored in the quantitative analysis.

Erythrocyte Count

Up to 20 years ago, blood cells were counted "by hand" in an optical counting chamber. This method has now been almost completely abandoned in favor of automated counters that determine the number of erythrocytes by measuring the impedance or light dispersion of EDTA blood (1 ml), or heparinized capillary blood. Due to differences in the hematocrit, the value from a sample taken after (at least 15 minutes') standing or physical activity will be 5–10% higher than the value from a sample taken after 15 minutes' bed rest.

Hemoglobin and Hematocrit Assay

Hemoglobin is oxidized to cyanmethemoglobin by the addition of cyanide, and the cyanmethemoglobin is then determined spectrophotometrically by the automated counter. The hematocrit describes the ratio of the volume of erythrocytes to the total blood volume (the SI unit is without dimension, e.g., 0.4).

The EDTA blood is centrifuged in a disposable capillary tube for 10 minutes using a high-speed microhematocrit centrifuge (reference method). The automated hematology counter determines the mean corpuscular or cell volume (MCV, measured in femtoliters, fl) and the number of erythrocytes. It calculates the hematocrit (HCT) using the following formula:

$$\text{HCT} = \text{MCV (fl)} \times \text{number of erythrocytes } (10^6/\mu l).$$

Calculation of Erythrocyte Parameters

The quality of erythrocytes is characterized by their MCV, their mean cell hemoglobin content (MCH), and the mean cellular hemoglobin concentration (MCHC).

MCV is measured directly using an automated hemoglobin analyzer, or is calculated as follows:

$$\text{MCV} = \frac{\text{Hematocrit (l/l)}}{\text{Number of erythrocytes } (10^6/\mu l)}$$

MCH (in picograms per erythrocyte) is calculated using the following formula:

$$\text{MCH (pg)} = \frac{\text{Hemoglobin (g/l)}}{\text{Number of erythrocytes } (10^6/\mu l)}$$

MCHC is determined using this formula:

$$\text{MCHC (g/dl)} = \frac{\text{Hemoglobin concentration (g/dl)}}{\text{Hematocrit (l/l)}}$$

Red Cell Distribution Width (RDW)

Modern analyzers also record the red cell distribution width (cell volume distribution). In normal erythrocyte morphology, this correlates with the Price-Jones curve for the cell diameter distribution. Discrepancies are used diagnostically and indicate the presence of microspherocytes (smaller cells with lighter central pallor).

Reticulocyte Count

Reticulocytes can be counted using flow cytometry and is based on the light absorbed by stained aggregates of reticulocyte organelles. The data are recorded as the number of reticulocytes per mill (‰) of the total number of erythrocytes. Reticulocytes can, of course, be counted in a counting chamber using a microscope. While this method is not particularly laborious, it is mostly employed in laboratories that often deal with or have a special interest in anemia. Reticulocytes are young erythrocytes immediately after they have extruded their nuclei: they contain, as a remainder of aggregated cell organelles, a net-like structure (hence the name "reticulocyte") that is not discernible after the usual staining procedures for leukocytes, but can be observed after vital staining of cells with brilliant cresyl blue or new methylene blue. The staining solution is mixed in an Eppendorf tube with an equal volume of EDTA blood and incubated for 30 minutes. After repeated mixing, a blood smear is prepared and allowed to dry. The sample is viewed using a microscope equipped with an oil immersion lens. The ratio of reticulocytes to erythrocytes is determined and plotted as reticulocytes per 1000 erythrocytes (per mill).

Normal values are listed in Table **2**, p. 12.

Table 2 Normal ranges and mean values for blood cell components*

		Adults > 18 years old	Newborns 1 months	Toddlers 2 years old	Children 10 years old
Leukocytes/µl or 10^6/l**	MV NR	**7000** 4300–10000	11000	10000	8000
Band granulocytes %	MV NR	**2** 0–5	5	3	3
Segmented neutrophilic granulocytes	MV NR	**60** 35–85	30	30	30
absolute ct./µl or 10^6/l**	MV NR	**3650** 1850–7250	3800	3500	4400
Lymphocytes %	MV NR	**30** 20–50	55	60	40
absolute ct./µl or 10^6/l**	MV NR	2500 **1500–3500**	6000	6300	3100
Monocytes %	MV NR	**4** 2–6	6	5	4
absolute ct./µl or 10^6/l**	MV NR	450 70–840			
Eosinophilic granulocytes (%)	MV NR	**2** 0–4	3	2	2
absolute ct./µl or 10^6/l**	MV NR	165 0–400			

Parameter	MV / NR	Male	Female			
Basophilic granulocytes (%)	MW / NR	**0.5** (0–1)		0.5	0.5	0.5
Erythrocytes $10^6/\mu l$ or $10^{12}/l$ [**]	MV / NR	**5.4** (4.6–5.9)	**4.8** (4.2–5.4)	4.7 (3.9–5.9)	4.7 (3.8–5.4)	4.8 (3.8–5.4)
Hb g/dl or 10 g/l [**]	MV / NR	**15** (14–18)	**13** (12–16)	17 (15–18)	12 (11–13)	14 (12–15)
HKT	MV / NR	**0.45** (0.42–0.48)	**0.42** (0.38–0.43)	44	37	39
MCH = Hb$_E$ (pg)	MV / NR	**29** (26–32)		33	27	25
MCV /μm^3 or fl [**]	MV / NR	**87** (77–99)		91	78	80
MCHC g/dl or 10 g/l	MV / NR	**33** (33–36)		35	33	34
Erythrocyte, diameter (μm)	MV	**7.5**		8.1	7.3	7.4
Reticulocytes (%)	MV / NR	**16** (8–25)	**24** (8–40)	7.9	7.1	7.6
Thrombocytes $10^3/\mu l$	MV / NR	**180** (140–440)		155–566	286–509	247–436

MV = mean value, NR = normal range (range for 95% of the population, reference range), ct. count. [**] SI units give the measurements per liter.
[*] For technical reasons, data may vary considerably between laboratories. It is therefore important also to consult the reference ranges of the chosen laboratory.

Leukocyte Count

Leukocytes, unlike erythrocytes, are completely colorless in their native state. Another important physical difference is the stability of leukocytes in 3% acetic acid or saponins; these media hemolyze erythrocytes (though not their nucleated precursors). Türk's solution, used in most counting methods, employs glacial acetic acid for hemolysis and crystal violet (gentian violet) to lightly stain the leukocytes. A 50-µl EDTA blood sample is mixed with 500 µl Türk's solution in an Eppendorf tube and incubated at room temperature for 10 minutes. The suspension is again mixed and carefully transferred to the well of a prepared counting chamber using a pipette or capillary tube. The chamber is allowed to fill from a droplet placed at one edge of the well and placed in a moisture-saturated incubator for 10 minutes. With the condenser lowered (or using phase contrast microscopy), the leukocytes are then counted in a total of four of the large squares opposite to each other (1 mm^2 each). The result is multiplied by 27.5 (dilution: 1 + 10, volume: 0.4 mm^3) to yield the leukocyte count per microliter. Parallel (control) counts show variation of up to 15%. The normal (reference) ranges are given in Table **2**.

In an automated blood cell counter, the erythrocytes are lysed and cells with a volume that exceeds about 30 fl (threshold values vary for different instruments) are counted as leukocytes. Any remaining erythroblasts, hard-to-lyse erythrocytes such as target cells, giant thrombocytes, or agglutinated thrombocytes are counted along with the leukocytes, and this will lead to an overestimate of the leukocyte count. Modern analyzers can recognize such interference factors and apply interference algorithms to obtain a corrected leukocyte count.

Visual leukocyte counts using a counting chamber show a variance of about 10%; they can be used as a control reference for automatic cell counts. Rough estimates can also be made by visual assessment of blood smears: a 40× objective will show an average of two to three cells per field of view if the leukocyte count is normal.

Thrombocyte Count

To count thrombocytes in a counting chamber, blood must be conditioned with 2% Novocain–Cl solution. Preprepared commercial tubes are widely used (e.g., Thrombo Plus with 2-ml content). EDTA blood is pipetted into the tubes, carefully mixed and immediately placed in a counting chamber. The chamber is allowed to stand for 10 minutes while the cells settle, after which an area of 1 mm^2 is counted. The result corresponds to the number of thrombocytes (the 1 + 100 dilution is ignored). In an automated blood cell counter, the blood cells are counted after they have been sorted by size. Small cells between 2 and 20 fl (thresholds vary for different instruments) are counted as thrombocytes. If giant thrombocytes or agglutinated thrombocytes are present, they are not counted and the result is an underestimate. On the other hand, small particles, such as fragmentocytes, or microcytes, will lead to an overestimate. Modern analyzers can recognize such interference factors and apply interference algorithms to obtain a corrected thrombocyte count. If unexpected results are produced, it is wise to check them by direct reference to the blood smear.

> **!** Unexpected thrombocyte counts should be verified by direct visual assessment. Using a 100× objective, the field of view normally contains an average of 10 thrombocytes. In some instances, "pseudothrombocytopenias" are found in automated counts. These are artifacts due to thrombocyte aggregation.

Pseudothrombocytopenia (see p. 167) is caused by the aggregation of thrombocytes in the presence of EDTA; it does not occur when heparin or citrate are used as anticoagulants.

Quantitative Normal Values and Range of Cellular Blood Components

Determining normal values for blood components is more difficult and more risky than one might expect. Obviously, the values are affected by a large number of variables, such as age, gender, activity (metabolic load), circadian rhythm, and nutrition, not to mention the effects of the blood sampling technique, type and storage of the blood, and the counting method. For this reason, where available, a normal *range* is given, covering 95% of the values found in a clinically normal group of probands—from which it follows that one in every 20 healthy people will have values outside the limits of this range. Thus, there are areas of overlap between normal and pathological data. Data in these borderline areas must be interpreted within a refined *reference range* with data from probands who resemble each other and the patient as closely as possible in respect of the variables listed above. Due to space limitations, only key age data are considered here. Figure **3** clearly shows that, particularly for newborns, toddlers, and young children, particular reference ranges must be taken into account. In addition, the interpretation must also take account of methodological variation: in cell counts, the coefficient of variation (standard deviation as a percentage of the mean value) is usually around 10!

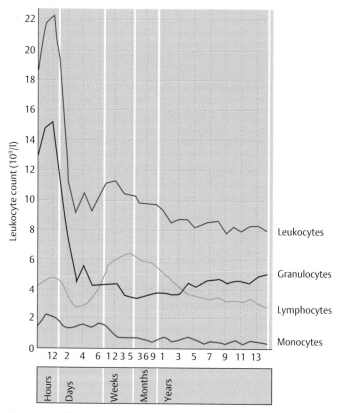

Fig. **3**   Mean cell counts at different ages in childhood for leukocytes and their subfractions (according to Kato)

> ❗ In sum, a healthy distrust for the single data point is the most important basis for the interpretation of all data, including those outside the reference range. For every sample of drawn blood, and every counting method, at least two or three values should be available before conclusions can be drawn, unless the clinical findings reflect the cytological data. In addition to this, every laboratory has its own set of reference data to some extent.

After this account of the problems and wide variations between different groups, the data in Table **2** are presented in a simplified form, with values rounded up or down for ease of comparison and memorization. Absolute values and the new SI units are given where they are clinically relevant.

The Blood Smear and Its Interpretation (Differential Blood Count, DBC)

A blood smear uses capillary or venous EDTA-blood, preferably no more than three hours old. The slides must be grease-free, otherwise cell aggregation and stain precipitation may occur. Unless commercially available grease-free slides are used, the slides should be soaked for several hours in a solution of equal parts of ethanol and ether and then allowed to dry. A droplet of the blood sample is placed close to the edge of the slide. A ground cover glass (spreader slide) is placed in front of the droplet onto the slide at an angle of about 30°. The cover slide is then slowly backed into the blood droplet. Upon contact, the blood droplet spreads along the edge of the slide (Fig. **4**). Without pressure, the cover glass is now lightly moved over the slide. The faster the cover glass is moved, and the steeper angle at which it is held, the thinner the smear will be.

> ❗ The quality of the smear technique is crucial for the assessment, because the cell density at the end of the smear is often twice that at the beginning.

In a well-prepared smear the blood sample will show a "feathered" edge where the cover glass left the surface of the slide. The smear must be thoroughly air-dried; for good staining, at least two hours' drying time is needed. The quality of the preparation will be increased by 10 minutes' fixation with methanol, and it will then also keep better. After drying, name and date are pencilled in on the slide.

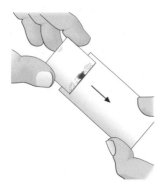

Fig. **4** Preparation of a blood smear

For safety's sake, at least one back-up smear should be made from every sample from every patient.

Staining is done with a mixture of basic stains (methylene blue, azure) and acidic stains (eosin), so as to show complementary substances such as nucleic acids and alkaline granulations. In addition to these leukocyte components, erythrocytes also yield different staining patterns: immature erythrocytes contain larger residual amounts of RNA and therefore stain more heavily with basophilic stains than do mature erythrocytes. Pappenheim's panoptic stain contains a balanced mixture of basic and acidic stains: the horizontally stored, air-dried smear is covered with May–Grünwald staining solution (eosin–methylene blue) for three minutes, then about an equal amount of phosphate buffer, pH = 7.3, is carefully added and, after a further three minutes, carefully poured off again. Next, the slide is covered with diluted Giemsa stain (azure–eosin), which is prepared by addition of 1 ml Giemsa stock solution to 1 ml neutral distilled water or phosphate buffer, pH = 6.8–7.4. After 15 minutes, the Giemsa staining solution is gently rinsed off with buffer solution and the smears are air-dried with the feathered end sloping upwards.

The blood smears are initially viewed with a smaller objective ($10\times$ to $20\times$), which allows the investigator to check the cell density and to find the best counting area in the smear. Experience shows that the cell projection is best about 1 cm from the feathered end of the smear. At $40\times$ magnification, one may expect to see an average of two to three leukocytes per viewing field if the leukocyte count is normal. It is sometimes useful to be able to use this rough estimate to crosscheck improbable quantitative values. The detailed analysis of the white blood cells is done using an oil immersion lens and $100\times$ magnification. For this, it is best to scan the section from about 1 cm to about 3 cm from the end of the smear, moving the slide to and fro in a meandering movement across its short diameter. Before (and while) the differential leukocyte count is carried out, erythrocyte morphology and thrombocyte density should be assessed. The results of the differential leukocyte count (the morphologies are presented in the atlas section, p. 30 ff.) may be recorded using manual counters or mark-up systems. The more cells are counted, the more representative the results, so when pathological deviations are found, it is advisable to count 200 cells.

To speed up the staining process, which can seem long and laborious when a rapid diagnosis is required, several quick-staining sets are available commercially, although most of them do not permit comparable fine analysis. If the standard staining solutions mentioned above are to hand, a quick stain for orientation purposes can be done by incubating the smear with May–Grünwald reagent for just one minute and shortening the Giemsa incubation time to one to two minutes with concentrated "solution."

Normal values and ranges for the differential blood count are given in Table **2**, p. 12.

Malaria plasmodia are best determined using a thick smear in addition to the normal blood smear. On a slide, a drop of blood is spread over an area of about 2.5 cm across. The thick smear is placed in an incubator and allowed to dry for at least 30 minutes. Drying samples as thick smears and then treating them with dilute Giemsa stain (as described above) achieves extensive hemolysis of the erythrocytes and thus an increase in the released plasmodia.

Significance of the Automated Blood Count

The qualitative and quantitative blood count techniques described here may seem somewhat archaic given the now almost ubiquitous automated cell counters; they are merely intended to show the possibilities always ready to be called on in terms of individual analyses carried out by small, dedicated laboratories.

The automated cell count has certainly rationalized blood cell counting. Depending on the diagnostic problem and the quality control system of the individual laboratory, automated counting can even reduce data ranges compared with "manual" counts.

After lysis of the erythrocytes, hematology analyzers determine the number of remaining nucleated cells using a wide range of technologies. All counters use cell properties such as size, interaction with scattered light at different angles, electrical conductivity, nucleus-to-cytoplasm ratio, and the peroxidase reaction, to group individual cell impulses into clusters. These clusters are then quantified and assigned to leukocyte populations.

If only normal blood cells are present, the assignment of the clusters to the various leukocyte populations works well, and the precision of the automated count exceeds that of the manual count of 100 cells in a smear by a factor of 10. If large number of pathological cells are present, such as blasts or lymphadenoma cells, samples are reliably recognized as "pathological," and a smear can then be prepared and further analyzed under the microscope.

The difficulty arises when small populations of pathological cells are present (e.g., 2% blasts present after chemotherapy), or when pathological cells are present that closely resemble normal leukocytes (e.g., small centrocytes in satellite cell lymphoma). These pathological conditions are not always picked up by automated analyzers (false negative result), no smear is prepared and studied under the microscope, and the results produced by the machine do not include the presence of these pathological populations. For this reason, blood samples accompanied by appropriate clinical queries (e.g., "lymphadenoma?" "blasts?" "unexplained anemia?") should always be differentiated and evaluated using a microscope.

Bone Marrow Biopsy

Occasionally, a disease of the blood cell system cannot be diagnosed and classified on the basis of the blood count alone and a bone marrow biopsy is indicated. In such cases it is more important to perform this biopsy competently and produce good smears for evaluation than to be able to interpret the bone marrow cytology yourself. Indications for bone marrow biopsy are given in Table **3**.

> In the attempt to avoid complications, the traditional location for bone marrow biopsy at the sternum has been abandoned in favor of the superior part of the posterior iliac spine (back of the hipbone) (Fig. **5**).

Although the **bone marrow cytology** findings from the aspirate are sufficient or even preferable for most hematological questions (see Table **3**), it is regarded as good practice to obtain a sample for **bone marrow histology** at the same time, since with improved instruments the procedure has become less stressful, and complementary cytological and histological data are then available from the start. After deep local anesthesia of the dorsal spine and a small skin incision, a histology cylinder at least 1.5 cm long is obtained using a sharp hollow needle (Yamshidi). A Klima and Rossegger cytology needle (Fig. **5**) is then placed through the same subcutaneous channel but at a slightly different site from the earlier insertion point on the spine and gently pushed through the compacta. The mandrel is pulled out and a 5- to 10-ml syringe body with 0.5 ml citrate or EDTA (heparin is used only for cytogenetics) is attached to the needle. The patient should be warned that there will be a painful drawing sensation during aspiration, which cannot be avoided. The barrel is then slowly pulled, and if the procedure is successful, blood from the bone marrow fills the syringe. The syringe body is separated from the needle and the mandrel reintroduced. The bone marrow aspirate is transferred from the syringe to a Petri dish. When the dish is gently shaken, small, pinhead-sized bone marrow spicules will be seen lying on the bottom. A smear, similar to a blood smear, can be prepared on a slide directly from the remaining contents of the syringe. If the first aspirate has obtained material, the needle is removed and a light compression bandage is applied.

If the aspirate for cytology contains no bone marrow fragments ("punctio sicca," dry tap), an attempt may be made to obtain a cytology smear from the (as yet unfixed) histology cylinder by rolling it carefully on the slide, but this seldom produces optimal results.

The preparation of the precious bone marrow material demands special care. One or two bone marrow spicules are pushed to the outer edge of the Petri dish, using the mandrel from the sternal needle, a needle, or a wooden rod with a beveled tip, and transferred to a fat-free microscopy slide, on which they are gently pushed to and fro by the needle along the length of the slide in a meandering line. This helps the analyzing

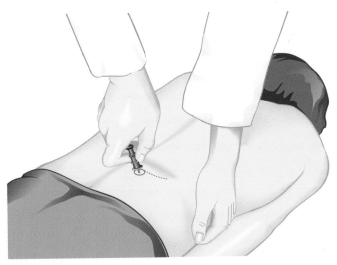

Fig. **5**   Bone marrow biopsy from the superior part of the posterior iliac spine (back of the hipbone)

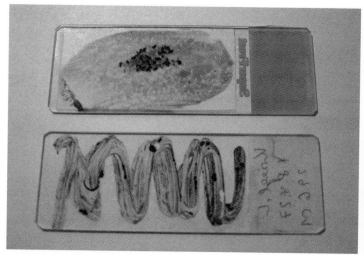

Fig. **6**   Squash preparation and meandering smear for the cytological analysis of bone marrow spicules

technician to make a differentiatial count. It should be noted that too much blood in the bone marrow sample will impede the semiquantitative analysis. In addition to this type of smear, squash preparations should also be prepared from the bone marrow material for selective staining. To do this, a few small pieces of bone marrow are placed on a slide and covered by a second slide. The two slides are lightly pressed and slid against each other, then separated (see Fig. **6**).

The smears are allowed to air-dry and some are incubated with panoptic Pappenheim staining solution (see previous text). Smears being sent to a diagnostic laboratory (wrapped individually and shipped as fragile goods) are better left unstained. Fresh smears of peripheral blood should accompany the shipment of each set of samples. (For principles of analysis and normal values see p. 52 ff., for indications for bone marrow cytology and histology see p. 27 ff.)

Lymph Node Biopsy and Tumor Biopsy

These procedures, less invasive than bone marrow biopsy, are a simple and often diagnostically sufficient method for lymph node enlargement or other intumescences. The unanesthetized, disinfected skin is sterilized and pulled taut over the node. A no. 1 needle on a syringe with good suction is pushed through the skin into the lymph node tissue (Fig. **7**). Tissue is aspirated from several locations, changing the angle of the needle slightly after each collection, and suction maintained while the needle is withdrawn into the subcutis. Aspiration ceases and the syringe is removed without suction. The biopsy harvest, which is in the needle, is extruded onto a microscopy slide and smeared out without force or pressure using a cover glass (spreader slide). Staining is done as described previously for blood smears.

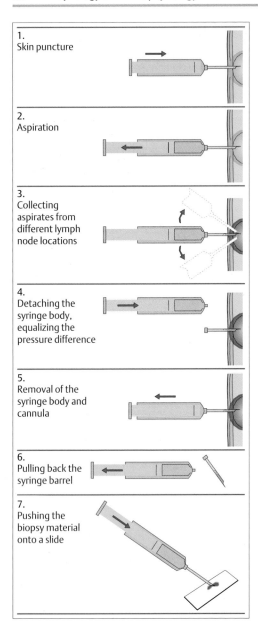

1.
Skin puncture

2.
Aspiration

3.
Collecting aspirates from different lymph node locations

4.
Detaching the syringe body, equalizing the pressure difference

5.
Removal of the syringe body and cannula

6.
Pulling back the syringe barrel

7.
Pushing the biopsy material onto a slide

Fig. **7**   Procedure for lymph node biopsy

Step-by-Step Diagnostic Sequence

On the basis of what has been said so far, the following guidelines for the diagnostic workup of hematological changes may be formulated:

1. The first step is *quantitative determination* of *leukocytes* (L), *erythrocytes* (E) and *thrombocytes* (T). Because the normal range can vary so widely in individual cases (Table **2**), the following rule of thumb should be observed:

> A complete blood count (CBC) should be included in the baseline data, like blood pressure.

2. All quantitative changes in L + E + T call for a careful *evaluation of the differential blood count* (DBC). Since clinical findings determine whether a DBC is indicated, it may be said that:

> A differential blood count is indicated:
> ➤ By all unexplained clinical symptoms, especially
> ➤ Enlarged lymph nodes or splenomegaly
> ➤ Significant changes in any of
>   – Hemoglobin content or number of erythrocytes
>   – Leukocyte count
>   – Thrombocyte count

The only initial assumption here is that *mononuclear cells* with unsegmented nuclei can be distinguished from *polynuclear cells*. While this nomenclature may not conform to ideal standards, it is well established and, moreover, of such practical importance as a fundamental distinguishing criterion that it is worth retaining. A marked majority of mononuclear cells over the polynuclear segmented granulocytes is an unambiguous early finding.

The next step has to be taken with far more care and discernment: *classifying the mononuclear cells according to their possible origin*, lymphatic cells, monocytes, or various immature blastic elements, which otherwise only occur in bone marrow. The aim of the images in the Atlas section of this book is to facilitate this part of the differential diagnosis. To a great extent, the possible origins of mononuclear cells can be distinguished; however, the limits of morphology and the vulnerability to artifacts are also apparent, leaving the door wide open to further diagnostic steps (specialist morphological studies, cytochemistry, immunocytochemistry. A predominance of mononuclear cell elements has the same critical significance in the differential diagnosis of both leukocytoses and leukopenias.

3. After the evaluation of the leukocytes, assessment of *erythrocyte morphology* is a necessary part of every blood smear evaluation. It is, naturally, particularly important in cases showing disturbances in the erythrocyte count or the hemoglobin.

4. After careful consideration of the results obtained so far and the patient's clinical record, the last step is the *analysis of the cell composition of the bone marrow*. Quite often, suspected diagnoses are confirmed through humoral tests such as electrophoresis, or through cytochemical tests such as alkaline phosphatase, myeloperoxidase, nonspecific esterase, esterase, or iron tests.

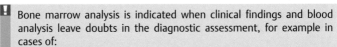

> Bone marrow analysis is indicated when clinical findings and blood analysis leave doubts in the diagnostic assessment, for example in cases of:
> - Leukocytopenia
> - Thrombocytopenia
> - Undefined anemia
> - Tricytopenia, or
> - Monoclonal hypergammaglobulinemia

A bone marrow analysis may be indicated in order to evaluate the spreading of a lymphadenoma or tumor, unless the bloodstream already shows the presence of pathological cells.

5. *Bone marrow histology* is also rarely indicated (even more rarely than the bone marrow cytology). Examples of the decision-making process between bone marrow cytology and histology (biopsy) are shown in Table **3**.

> Often only histological analysis can show structural changes or focal infiltration of the bone marrow.

This is particularly true of the frequently fiber-rich chronic myeloproliferative diseases, such as polycythemia vera rubra, myelofibrosis–osteomyelosclerosis (MF-OMS), essential thrombocythemia (ET), and chronic myeloid leukemia (CML) as well as *malignant lymphoma* without hematological involvement (Hodgkin disease or blastic non-Hodgkin lymphoma) and *tumor infiltration*.

Table **3** Indications for a differential blood count (DBC), bone marrow aspiration, and biopsy

Indications	Procedures	
All clinically unclear situations: ➤ Enlarged lymph nodes or spleen ➤ Changes in the simple CBC (penias or cytoses)	Differential blood count (DBC)	
➤ When a diagnosis cannot be made based on clinical findings and analysis of peripheral blood differential blood analysis, cytochemistry, phenotyping, molecular genetics or FISH	Bone marrow analysis	
	Bone marrow aspirate (Morphology, phenotyping, cytogenetics, FISH, molecular genetics)	**Bone marrow trephine biopsy** (Morphology, immuno-histology)
➤ Punctio sicca ("dry tap")	not possible	+
➤ Aplastic bone marrow	not possible	+
➤ Suspicion of myelodysplastic syndrome	+	(+) (e.g. hypoplasia)
➤ Pancytopenia	+	+
➤ Anemia, isolated	+	–
➤ Granulocytopenia, isolated	+	–
➤ Thrombocytopenia, isolated (except ITP)	+	–
➤ Suspected ITP	(+) For therapy failure	–
➤ Suspected OMF/OMS	– (*BCR-ABL* in peripheral blood is sufficient)	+
➤ Suspected PV	– (*BCR-ABL* in peripheral blood is sufficient)	–
➤ Suspected ET	– (*BCR-ABL* in peripheral blood is sufficient)	+
➤ Suspected CML	– (*BCR-ABL* in peripheral blood is sufficient)	(+) Conditions for the analysis
➤ CMPE (*BCR-ABL* negative)	(+) Differential diagnoses	+
➤ Suspected AL/AL	+	(+) Not in typical cases
➤ Suspected bone marrow metastases	–	+
➤ Monoclonal hypergammaglobulinemia	+	+
➤ NHL (exceptions, see below)	+	+
➤ Typical CLL	+	(+) Prognostic factor
➤ Follicular lymphoma	(+) To distinguish vs other NHL	+
➤ Hodgkin disease	–	+
Further indications for a bone marrow analysis are:		
➤ Unexplained hypercalcemia	+	+
➤ Inexplicable increase of bone AP	–	+
➤ Obvious, unexplained abnormalities	–	+
➤ Hyperparathyroidism	–	+
➤ Paget disease	–	+
➤ Osteomalacia	–	+
➤ Renal osteopathy	–	+
➤ Gaucher syndrome	–	+

+ Recommended, – not recommended, (+) conditionally recommended, ITP idiopathic thrombocytopenia, OMF/OMS osteomyelofibrosis/osteomyelosclerosis, PV polycythemia vera, ET essential thrombocythemia, CMPD chronic myeloproliferative disorders, AL acute leukemia, NHL non-Hodgkin lymphoma, CLL chronic lymphocytic leukemia, FISH fluorescence in situ hybridization, AP alkaline phosphatase.

Normal Cells of the Blood and Hematopoietic Organs

The Individual Cells of Hematopoiesis

Immature Red Cell Precursors: Proerythroblasts and Basophilic Erythroblasts

Proerythroblasts are the earliest, least mature cells in the erythrocyte-forming series (erythropoiesis). Proerythroblasts are characterized by their size (about 20 μm), and by having a very dense nuclear structure with a narrow layer of cytoplasm, homogeneous in appearance, with a lighter zone at the center; they stain deep blue after Romanowsky staining. These attributes allow proerythroblasts to be distinguished from myeloblasts (p. 35) and thus to be assigned to the erythrocyte series. After mitosis, their daughter cells display similar characteristics except that they have smaller nuclei. Daughter cells are called *basophilic erythroblasts* (formerly also called *macroblasts*). Their nuclei are smaller and the chromatin is more coarsely structured.

The maturation of cells in the erythrocyte series is closely linked to the activity of macrophages (transformed monocytes), which phagocytose nuclei expelled from normoblasts and iron from senescent erythrocytes, and pass these cell components on to developing erythrocytes.

Diagnostic Implications. Proerythrocytes exist in circulating blood only under pathological conditions (extramedullary hematopoiesis; breakdown of the blood–bone marrow barrier by tumor metastases, p. 150; or erythroleukemia, p. 100). In these situations, basophilic erythroblasts may also occur; only exceptionally in the course of a strong postanemia regeneration will a very few of these be released into the blood stream (e.g., in the compensation phase after severe hemorrhage or as a response to vitamin deficiency, see p. 152).

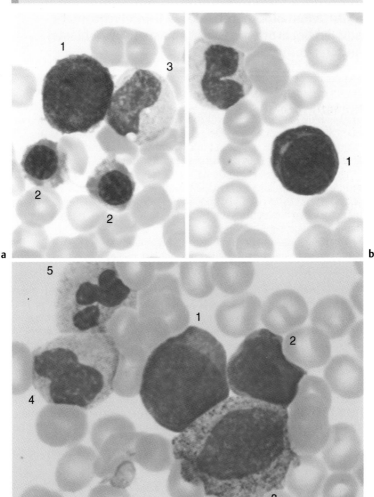

Fig. 8 Early erythropoiesis. **a** The earliest recognizable red cell precursor is the large dark proerythroblast with loosely arranged nuclear chromatin (1). Below are two orthochromatic erythroblasts (2), on the right a metamyelocyte (3). **b** Pro-erythroblast (1). **c** Proerythroblast (1) next to a myeloblast (2) (see p. 34); lower region of image shows a promyelocyte (3). Toward the upper left are a metamyelocyte (4) and a segmented neutrophilic granulocyte (5).

Mature Red Blood Precursor Cells: Polychromatic and Orthochromatic Erythroblasts (Normoblasts) and Reticulocytes

The results of mitosis of erythroblasts are called *normoblasts*. This name covers two cell types with relatively dense round nuclei and grayish pink stained cytoplasm. The immature cells in which the cytoplasm displays a grayish blue hue, which are still able to divide, are now called "polychromatic erythroblasts," while the cells in which the cytoplasm is already taking on a pink hue, which contain a lot of hemoglobin and are no longer able to divide, are called "orthochromatic erythroblasts." The nuclei of the latter gradually condense into small black spheres without structural definition that eventually are expelled from the cells. The now enucleated young erythrocytes contain copious ribosomes that precipitate into reticular ("net-like") structures after special staining (see p. 11), hence their name, *reticulocytes.*

To avoid confusing erythroblasts and lymphoblasts (Fig. **9 d**), note the completely rounded, very dense normoblast nuclei and homogeneous, unstructured cytoplasm of the erythroblasts.

Diagnostic Implications. Polychromatic and orthochromatic erythroblasts may be released into the bloodstream whenever hematopoiesis is activated, e.g., in the compensation or treatment stage after hemorrhage or iron or vitamin deficiency. They are always present when turnover of blood cells is chronically increased (hemolysis). Once increased blood regeneration has been excluded, the presence of erythroblasts in the blood should prompt consideration of two other disorders: extramedullary production of blood cells in myeloproliferative diseases (p. 114), and bone marrow carcinosis with destruction of the blood–bone marrow barrier (p. 154). In the same situations, the reticulocyte counts (after special staining) are elevated above the average of 25‰ for men and 40‰ for women, respectively, and can reach extremes of several hundred per mill.

Fig. **9**   Nucleated erythrocyte precursors. **a** Two basophilic erythroblasts with ▶ condensed chromatin structure (1) and a polychromatic erythroblast with an almost homogeneous nucleus (2). **b** The erythropoiesis in the bone marrow is often organized around a macrophage with a very wide, light cytoplasmic layer (1). Grouped around it are polychromatic erythroblasts of variable size. Erythroblast mitosis (2). **c** Polychromatic erythroblast (1) and orthochromatic erythroblast (normoblast) (2).

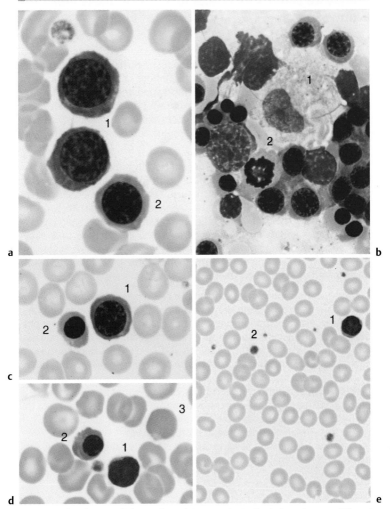

Fig. **9** **d** The density of the nuclear chromatin is similar in lymphocytes (1) and erythroblasts (2), but in the erythroblast the cytoplasm is wider and similar in color to a polychromatic erythrocyte (3). **e** Normal red blood cell findings with slight variance in size of the erythrocytes. A lymphocyte (1) and a few thrombocytes (2) are seen. The erythrocytes are slightly smaller than the nucleus of the lymphocyte nucleus.

Immature White Cell Precursors: Myeloblasts and Promyelocytes

Myeloblasts are the least mature cells in the granulocyte lineage. Mononuclear, round-to-ovoid cells, they may be distinguished from proerythroblasts by the finer, "grainy" reticular structure of their nuclei and the faintly basophilic cytoplasm. On first impression, they may look like large or even small lymphocytes (micromyeloblasts), but the delicate structure of their nuclei always gives them away as myeloblasts. In some areas, condensed chromatin may start to look like nucleoli. Sporadically, the cytoplasm contains azurophilic granules.

Promyelocytes are the product of myeloblast division, and usually grow larger than their progenitor cells. During maturation, their nuclei show an increasingly coarse chromatin structure. The nucleus is eccentric; the lighter zone over its bay-like indentation corresponds to the Golgi apparatus. The wide layer of basophilic cytoplasm contains copious large azurophilic granules containing peroxidases, hydrolases, and other enzymes. These granulations also exist scattered all around the nucleus, as may be seen by focusing on different planes of the preparation using the micrometer adjustment on the microscope.

Diagnostic Implications. Ordinarily, both cell types are encountered only in the bone marrow, where they are the most actively dividing cells and main progenitors of granulocytes. In times of increased granulocyte production, promyelocytes and (in rare cases) myeloblasts may be released into the blood stream (pathological left shift, see p. 112). Under strong regeneration pressure from the erythrocyte series, too—e.g., during the compensation phase following various anemias—immature white cell precursors, like the red cell precursors, may be swept into the peripheral blood. Bone marrow involvement by tumor metastases also increases the permeability of the blood–bone marrow barrier for immature white cell precursors (for an overview, see p. 112 ff.).

In some acute forms of leukemia, myeloblasts (and also, rarely, promyelocytes) dominate the blood analysis (p. 97).

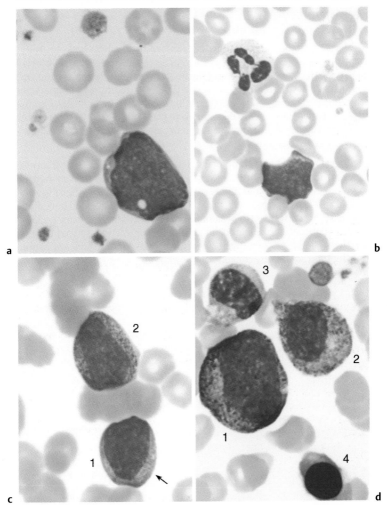

Fig. **10** Granulocyte precursors. **a** The least mature precursor in granulopoiesis is the myeloblast, which is released into the blood stream only under pathological conditions. A large myeloblast is shown with a fine reticular nuclear structure and a narrow layer of slightly basophilic cytoplasm without granules. **b** Myeloblast and neutrophilic granulocytes with segmented nuclei (blood smear from a patient with AML). **c** Myeloblast (1), which shows the start of azurophilic granulation (arrow), and a promyelocyte (2) with copious large azurophilic granules, typically in a perinuclear location. **d** Large promyelocyte (1), myelocyte (2), metamyelocyte (3), and polychromatic erythroblast (4).

35

Partly Mature White Cell Precursors: Myelocytes and Metamyelocytes

Myelocytes are the direct product of promyelocyte mitosis and are always clearly smaller than their progenitors. The ovoid nuclei have a banded structure; the cytoplasm is becoming lighter with maturation and in some cases acquiring a pink tinge. A special type of granules, which no longer stain red like the granules in promyelocytes ("specific granules," peroxidase-negative), are evenly distributed in the cytoplasm. Myelocyte morphology is wide-ranging because myelocytes actually cover three different varieties of dividing cells.

Metamyelocytes (*young* granulocytes) are the product of the final myelocyte division and show further maturation of the nucleus with an increasing number of stripes and points of density that give the nuclei a spotted appearance. The nuclei slowly take on a kidney bean shape and have some plasticity. Metamyelocytes are unable to divide. From this stage on, only further maturation of the nucleus occurs by contraction, so that the distinctions (between metamyelocytes, band neutrophils, and segmented neutrophils) are merely conventional, although they do relate to the varying "maturation" of these cell forms.

Diagnostic Implications. Like their precursors, myelocytes and metamyelocytes normally appear in the peripheral blood only during increased cell production in response to stress or triggers, especially infections (for an overview of possible triggers, see p. 112). Under these conditions, they are, however, more abundant than myeloblasts or promyelocytes.

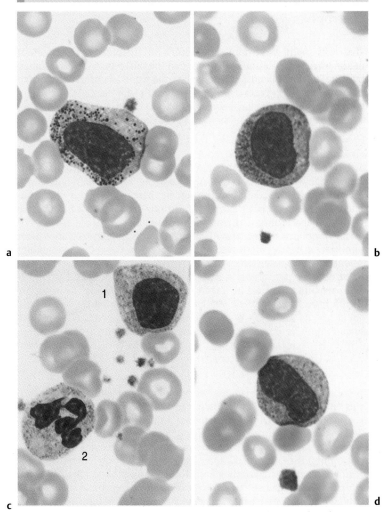

Fig **11** Myelocytes and metamyelocytes. **a** Early myelocyte. The chromatin structure is denser than that of promyelocytes. The granules do not lie over the nucleus (as can be seen by turning the fine focus adjustment of the microscope to and fro). The blood smear is from a case of sepsis, hence the intensive granulation. **b** Slightly activated myelocyte (the cytoplasm is still relatively basophilic). **c** Typical myelocyte (1) close to a segmented neutrophil (2). **d** This metamyelocyte is distinguished from a myelocyte by incipient lobe formation.

Mature Neutrophils: Band Cells and Segmented Neutrophils

Band cells (band neutrophils) represent the further development of metamyelocytes. Distinguishing between the different cell types is often difficult. The term "band cell" should be used when all nuclear sections of the nucleus are approximately the same width (the "bands"). The beginnings of segmentation may be visible, but the indentations should never cut more than two-thirds of the way across the nucleus.

Segmented neutrophils represent the final stage in the lineage that started with myeloblasts, forming gradually, without any clear transition or further cell divisions, by increasing contraction of their nuclei. Finally, the nuclear segments are connected only by narrow chromatin bridges, which should be no thicker than one-third of the average diameter of the nucleus. The chromatin in each segment forms coarse bands, or patches, and is denser than the chromatin in band neutrophils.

The cytoplasm of segmented neutrophilic granulocytes varies after staining from nearly colorless to soft pink or violet. The abundant granules are often barely visible dots.

The number of segments increases with the age of the cells. The following approximate values are taken to represent a normal distribution: 10–30% have two segments, 40–50% have three segments, 10–20% have four segments, and 0–5% of the nuclei have five segments. A left shift to smaller numbers of segments is a discreet symptom of reactive activation of this cell series. A right shift to higher numbers of segments (oversegmentation) usually accompanies vitamin B_{12} and folic acid deficiencies.

Diagnostic Implications. *Banded* neutrophilic granulocytes (band neutrophils) may occur in small numbers (up to 2%) in a normal blood count. This is of no diagnostic significance. A higher proportion than 2% may indicate a left shift and constitute the first sign of a reactive condition (p. 113). The diagnostic value of *segmented* neutrophilic granulocytes (segmented neutrophils) is that normal values are the most sensitive diagnostic indicator of normally functioning hematopoiesis (and, especially, of normal cellular defense against bacteria). An increase in segmented neutrophils without a qualitative left shift is not evidence of an alteration in bone marrow function, because under certain conditions stored cells may be released into the peripheral blood (for causes, see p. 111). In conjunction with qualitative changes (left shift, toxic granulations), however, granulocytosis does in fact indicate bone marrow activation that may have a variety of triggers (pp. 110 f.), and if the absolute number has fallen below the lower limit of the normal range (Table **2**, p. 12), a bone marrow defect or increased cell death must be considered.

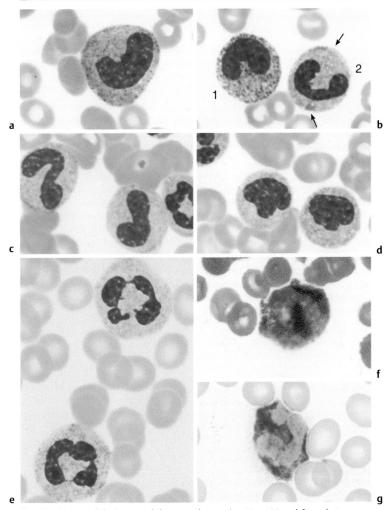

Fig. 12 Neutrophils (neutrophilic granulocytes). a Transitional form between a metamyelocyte and a band cell. b Copious granulation in a band cell (1) (toxic granulation) next to band cells (2) with Döhle bodies (arrows). c Two band cells. d Band cells can also occur as aggregates. e Segmented neutrophilic granulocytes. f Segmented neutrophilic granulocyte after the peroxidase reaction. g Segmented neutrophilic granulocyte after alkaline leukocyte phosphatase (ALP) staining.

39

Cell Degradation, Special Granulations, and Nuclear Appendages in Neutrophilic Granulocytes and Nuclear Anomalies

Toxic granulation is the term used when the normally faint stippled granules in segmented neutrophils stain an intense reddish violet, usually against a background of slightly basophilic cytoplasm; unlike the normal granules, they stain particularly well in an acidic pH (5.4). This phenomenon is a consequence of activity against bacteria or proteins and is observed in serious infections, toxic or drug effects, or autoimmune processes (e.g., chronic polyarthritis). At the same time, cytoplasmic *vacuoles* are often found, representing the end stage of phagocytosis (especially in cases of sepsis), as are Döhle bodies: small round bodies of basophilic cytoplasm that have been described particularly in scarlet fever, but may be present in all serious infections and toxic conditions. A deficiency or complete absence of granulation in neutrophils is a sign of severe disturbance of the maturation process (e.g., in myelodysplasia or acute leukemia). The *Pelger anomaly*, named after its first describer, is a hereditary segmentation anomaly of granulocytes that results in round, rod-shaped, or bisegmented nuclei. The same appearance as a nonhereditary condition (pseudo-Pelger formation, also called Pel–Ebstein fever, or [cyclic] Murchison syndrome) indicates a severe infectious or toxic stress response or incipient myelodysplasia; it also may accompany manifest leukemia.

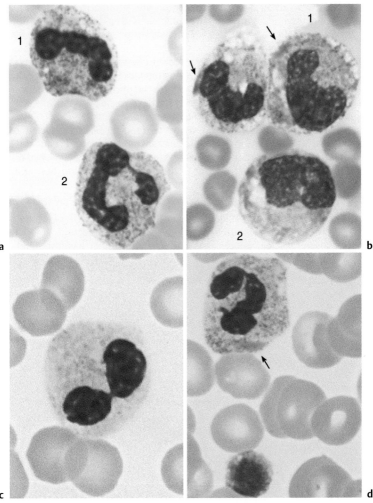

Fig. **13** Variations of segmented neutrophilic granulocytes. **a** Reactive state with toxic granulation of the neutrophilic granulocytes, more visibly expressed in the cell on the left (1) than the cell on the right (2) (compare with nonactivated cells, p. 39). **b** Sepsis with toxic granulation, cytoplasmic vacuoles, and Döhle bodies (arrows) in band cells (1) and a monocyte (2). **c** Pseudo-Pelger cell looking like sunglasses (toxic or myelodysplastic cause). **d** Döhle-like basophilic inclusion (arrow) without toxic granulation. Together with giant thrombocytes this suggests May–Hegglin anomaly. *continued* ▶

Nuclear appendages, which must not to be mistaken for small segments, are minute (less than the size of a thrombocyte) chromatin bodies that remain connected to the main part of the nucleus via a thin bridge and consequently look like a drumstick, sessile nodule, or small tennis racket. Of these, only the drumstick form corresponds to the X-chromosome, which has become sequestered during the process of segmentation. A proportion of 1–5% circulating granulocytes with drumsticks (at least 6 out of 500) suggests female gender; however, because the drumstick form is easy to confuse with the other (insignificant) forms of nuclear appendage, care should be taken before jumping to conclusions.

Rarely, *degrading forms* of granulocytes, shortly before cytolysis or apoptosis, may be found in the blood (they are more frequent in exudates). In these, the segments of the nucleus are clearly losing connection, and the chromatin structure of the individual segments, which are becoming round, becomes dense and homogeneous.

Diagnostic Implications. *Toxic granulation* indicates bacterial, chemical, or metabolic stress. *Pseudo-Pelger* granulocytes are observed in cases of infectious–toxic stress conditions, myelodysplasia, and leukemia.

The use of nuclear appendages to determine gender has lost significance in favor of genetic testing.

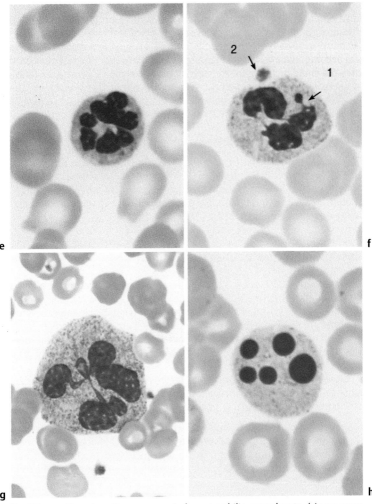

Fig. **13** continued. **e** Hypersegmented neutrophilic granulocyte (six or more segments). There is an accumulation of these cells in megaloblastic anemia. **f** Drumstick (arrow 1) as an appendage with a thin filament bridge to the nucleus (associated with the X-chromosome), adjoined by a thrombocyte (arrow 2). **g** Very large granulocyte from a blood sample taken after chemotherapy. **h** Segmented neutrophilic granulocyte during degradation, often seen as an artifact after prolonged sample storage (more than eight hours).

43

Eosinophilic Granulocytes (Eosinophils)

Eosinophils arise from the same stem cell population as neutrophils and mature in parallel with them. The earliest point at which eosinophils can be morphologically defined in the bone marrow is at the promyelocyte stage. Promyelocytes contain large granules that stain blue–red; not until they reach the metamyelocyte stage do these become a dense population of increasingly round, golden-red granules filling the cytoplasm. The Charcot–Leyden crystals found between groups of eosinophils in exudates and secretions have the same chemical composition as the eosinophil granules.

The nuclei of mature eosinophils usually have only two segments.

Diagnostic Implications. In line with their function (see p. 5) (reaction against parasites and regulation of the immune response, especially defense against foreign proteins), an increase of eosinophils above 400/μl should be seen as indicating the presence of parasitosis, allergies, and many other conditions (p. 124).

Basophilic Granulocytes (Basophils)

Like eosinophils, basophils (basophilic granulocytes) mature in parallel with cells of the neutrophil lineage. The earliest stage at which they can be identified is the promyelocyte stage, at which large, black–violet stained granules are visible. In mature basophils, which are relatively small, these granules often overlie the two compact nuclear segments like blackberries. However, they easily dissolve in water, leaving behind faintly pink stained vacuoles.

Close relations of basophilic granulocytes are tissue basophils or tissue mast cells—but these are never found in blood. Tissue basophils have a round nucleus underneath large basophilic granules.

Diagnostic Implications. In line with their role in anaphylactic reactions (p. 5), elevated basophil counts are seen above all in hypersensitivity reactions of various kinds. Basophils are also increased in chronic myeloproliferative bone marrow diseases, especially chronic myeloid leukemia (pp. 117, 120).

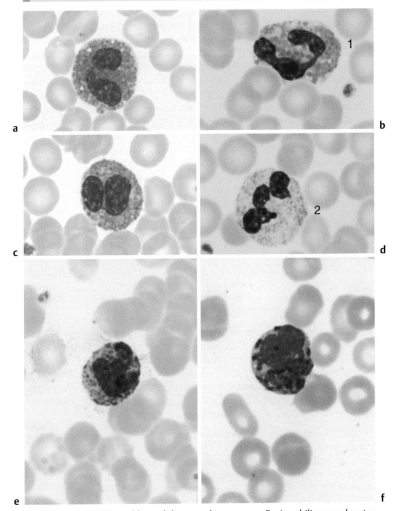

Fig. **14** Eosinophilic and basophilic granulocytes. **a–c** Eosinophilic granulocytes with corpuscular, orange-stained granules. **d** In contrast, the granules of neutrophilic granulocytes are not round but more bud-shaped. **e** Basophilic granulocyte. The granules are corpuscular like those of the eosinophilic granulocyte but stain deep blue to violet. **f** Very prominent large granules in a basophilic granulocyte in chronic myeloproliferative disease.

Monocytes

Monocytes are produced in the bone marrow; their line of development branches off at a very early stage from that of the granulocytic series (see flow chart p. **3**), but does not contain any distinct, specific precursors that can be securely identified with diagnostic significance in everyday morphological studies. Owing to their great motility and adhesiveness, mature monocytes are morphologically probably the most diversified of all cells. Measuring anywhere between 20 and 40 μm in size, their constant characteristic is an ovoid nucleus, usually irregular in outline, with invaginations and often pseudopodia-like cytoplasmic processes. The fine, "busy" structure of their nuclear chromatin allows them to be distinguished from myelocytes, whose chromatin has a patchy, streaky structure, and also from lymphocytes, which have dense, homogeneous nuclei. The basophilic cytoplasmic layer varies in width, stains a grayish color, and contains a scattered population of very fine reddish granules that are at the very limit of the eye's resolution. These characteristics vary greatly with the size of the monocyte, which in turn is dependent on the thickness of the smear. Where the smear is thin, especially at the feathered end, monocytes are abundant, relatively large and loosely structured, and their cytoplasm stains light gray–blue ("dove gray"). In thick, dense parts of the smear, some monocytes look more like lymphocytes: only a certain nuclear indentation and the "thundercloud" gray–blue staining of the cytoplasm may still mark them out.

Diagnostic Implications. In line with their function (see p. 5) as phagocytic defense cells, an elevation of the monocyte population above 7% and above 850/μl indicates an immune defense reaction; only when a sharp rise in monocyte counts is accompanied by a drop in absolute counts in the other cell series is monocytic leukemia suggested (p. 101). Phagocytosis of erythrocytes and white blood cells (hemophagocytosis) may occur in some virus infections and autoimmune diseases.

➤ Monocytosis in cases of *infection:* always present at the end of acute infections; chronic especially in
  – Endocarditis lenta, listeriosis, brucellosis, tuberculosis
➤ Monocytosis in cases of a *non-infectious response*, e.g.,
  – Collagenosis, Crohn disease, ulcerative colitis
➤ Monocytoses in/as *neoplasia*, e.g.,
  – Paraneoplastic in cases of disseminating tumors, bronchial carcinoma, breast carcinoma, Hodgkin disease, myelodysplasias (especially CMML, pp. 107 f) and acute monocytic leukemia (p. 101)

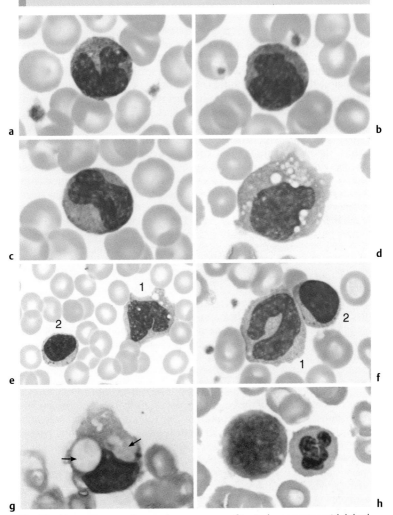

Fig. 15 **Monocytes. a–c** Range of appearances of typical monocytes with lobed, nucleus, gray–blue stained cytoplasm and fine granulation. **d** Phagocytic monocyte with plasma vacuoles. **e** Monocyte (1) to the right of a lymphocyte with azurophilic granules (2). **f** Monocyte (1) with nucleus resembling that of a band neutrophil, but its cytoplasm stains typically gray–blue. Lymphocyte (2). **g** A monocyte that has phagocytosed two erythrocytes and harbors them in its wide cytoplasm (arrows) (sample taken after bone marrow transplantation). **h** Esterase staining, a typical marker enzyme for cells of the monocyte lineage.

Lymphocytes (and Plasma Cells)

Lymphocytes are produced everywhere, particularly in the lymph nodes, spleen, bone marrow, and the lymphatic islands of the intestinal mucosa, under the influence of the thymus (T-lymphocytes, about 80%), or the bone marrow (B-lymphocytes, about 20%). A small fraction of the lymphocytes are NK cells (natural killer cells). Immature precursor cells (lymph node cytology, p. 177) are practically never released into the blood and are therefore of no practical diagnostic significance. The cells encountered in circulating blood are mostly "small" lymphocytes with oval or round nuclei 6–9 μm in diameter. Their chromatin may be described as dense and coarse. Detailed analysis under the microscope, using the micrometer screw to view the chromatin in different planes, reveals not the patch-like or banded structure of myeloblast chromatin, or the "busy" structure of monocyte chromatin, but slate-like formations with homogeneous chromatin and intermittent narrow, lighter layers that resemble geological break lines. Nucleoli are rarely seen. The cytoplasm wraps quite closely around the nucleus and is slightly basophilic. Only a few lymphocytes display the violet stained stippling of granules; about 5% of *small* lymphocytes and about 3% of *large* ones. The family of large lymphocytes with granulation consists mostly of NK cells. An important point is that small lymphocytes—which cannot be identified as T- or B-lymphocytes on the basis of morphology—are not functional end forms, but undergo transformation in response to specific immunological stimuli. The final stage of B-lymphocyte maturation (in bone marrow and lymph nodes) is plasma cells, whose nuclei often show radial bars, and whose basophilic cytoplasm layer is always wide. Intermediate forms ("plasmacytoid" lymphocytes) also exist.

Diagnostic Implications. Values between 1500 and 4000/μl and about 35% reflect normal output of the lymphatic system. Elevated absolute lymphocyte counts, often along with cell transformation, are observed predominantly in viral infections (pp. 67, 69) or in diseases of the lymphatic system (p. 75 ff.). Relative increases at the expense of other blood cell series may be a manifestation of toxic or aplastic processes (agranulocytosis, p. 87; aplastic anemia, p. 148), because these irregularities are rare in the lymphatic series. A spontaneous decrease in lymphocyte counts is normally seen only in very rare congenital diseases (agammaglobulinemia [Bruton disease], DiGeorge disease [chromosome 22q11 deletion syndrome]). Some systemic diseases also lead to low lymphocyte counts (Hodgkin disease, active AIDS).

Mature plasma cells are rarely found in blood (plasma cell leukemia is extremely rare). Plasma-cell-like ("plasmacytoid") lymphocytes occur in viral infections or systemic diseases (see p. 68 f. and p. 74 f.).

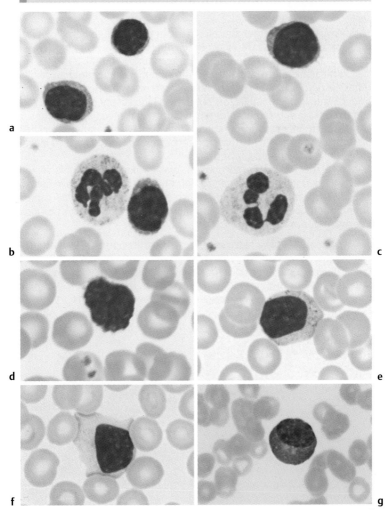

Fig. **16** Lymphocytes **a–c** Range of appearance of normal lymphocytes (some of them adjacent to segmented neutrophilic granulocytes). **d** In neonates, some lymphocytes from a neonate show irregularly shaped nuclei with notches or hints of segmentation. **e** A few larger lymphocytes with granules may occur in a normal person. **f** Occasionally, and without any recognizable trigger, the cytoplasm may widen. **g** A smear taken after infection may contain a few plasma cells, the final, morphologically fully developed cells in the B-lymphocyte series (for further activated lymphocyte forms, see p. 67).

49

Megakaryocytes and Thrombocytes

Megakaryocytes can enter the bloodstream only in highly pathological myeloproliferative disease or acute leukemia. They are shown here in order to demonstrate thrombocyte differentiation. Megakaryocytes reside in the bone marrow and have giant, extremely hyperploid nuclei (16 times the normal number of chromosome sets on average), which build up by endomitosis. Humoral factors regulate the increase of megakaryocytes and the release of thrombocytes when more are needed (e.g., bleeding or increased thrombocyte degradation). Cytoplasm with granules is pinched off from megakaryocytes to form thrombocytes. The residual naked megakaryocyte nuclei are phagocytosed.

Only mature *thrombocytes* occur in blood. About 1–4 μm in size and anuclear, their light blue stained cytoplasm and its processes give them a star-like appearance, with fine reddish blue granules near the center. Young thrombocytes are larger and more "spread out;" older ones look like pyknotic dots.

Diagnostic Implications. In a blood smear, there are normally 8–15 thrombocytes per view field using a 100× objective; they may appear dispersed or in groups. To someone quickly screening a smear, they will give a good indication of any increase or strong decrease in the count, which can be useful for early diagnosis of acute thrombocytopenias (p. 164 f.).

Small megakaryocyte nuclei are found in the bloodstream only in severe myeloproliferative disorders (p. 171).

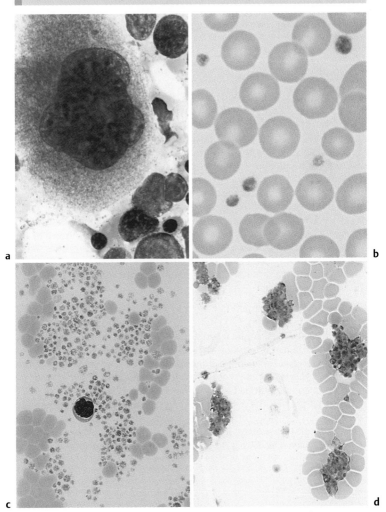

Fig. **17** Megakaryocytes and thrombocytes. **a** Megakaryocytes in a bone marrow smear. The wide cytoplasm displays fine, cloudy granulation as a sign of incipient thrombocyte budding. **b** Normal density of thrombocytes among the erythrocytes, with little variation in thrombocyte size. **c** and **d** Peripheral blood smears with aggregations of thrombocytes. When such aggregates are seen against a background of apparent thrombocytopenia, the phenomenon is called "pseudo-thrombocytopenia" and is usually an effect of the anticoagulant EDTA (see also p. 167).

51

Bone Marrow: Cell Composition and Principles of Analysis

As indicated above, and as will be shown below, almost all disorders of the hematopoietic system can be diagnosed using clinical findings, blood analysis, and humoral data. There is no mystery about bone marrow diagnostics. The basic categories are summarized here to give an understanding of how specific diagnostic information is achieved; photomicrographs will show the appearance of specific diseases. Once the individual cell types, as given in the preceding pages, are recognized, it becomes possible to interpret the bone marrow smears that accompany the various diseases, and to follow further, analogous diagnostic steps. As a first step in the analysis of a bone marrow tissue smear or squash preparation, various areas in several preparations are broadly surveyed. This is followed by individual analysis of at least 200 cells from two representative areas. Table **4** shows the mean normal values and their wide ranges.

A combination of estimation and quantitative analysis is used, based on the following criteria:

Cell Density. This parameter is very susceptible to artifacts. Figure **18** shows roughly the normal cell density. A lower count may be due to the manner in which the sample was obtained or to the smearing procedure. A bone marrow smear typically shows areas where connective tissue adipocytes with large vacuoles predominate. Only if these adipocytes areas are present is it safe to assume that the smear contains bone marrow material and that an apparent deficit of bone marrow cells is real.

Increased cell density: e.g., in all strong regeneration or compensation processes, and in cases of leukemia and myeloproliferative syndromes (except osteomyelosclerosis).

Decreased cell density: e.g., in aplastic processes and myelofibrosis.

Table **4** Cell composition in the bone marrow: normal values (%)

	Median values (J. Boll)	Median values and normal range (K. Rohr)	
Red cell series			
– Proerythrocytes	1		
– Macroblasts (basophilic erythroblasts)	3	3.5	0.5–7.5
– Normoblasts (poly- and orthochromic erythroblasts)	16	19	(7–40)
Neutrophil series			
– Myeloblasts	2.7	1	(0.5–5)
– Promyelocytes	9.5	3	(0–7.5)
– Myelocytes	14	15	(5–25)
– Metamyelocytes	10.5	15	(5–20)
– Band neutrophils	9.8	15	(5–25)
– Segmented neutrophils	17.5	7	(0.5–15)
Small cell series			
– Eosinophilic granulocytes	5	3	(1–7)
– Basophilic granulocytes	1	0.5	(0–1)
– Monocytes	2	2	(0.5–3)
– Lymphocytes	6	7.5	(2.5–15)
– Plasma cells	1.5	1	(0.5–3)

Megakaryocytes
Cell densities vary widely, 0.5–2 per view field during screening at low magnification.

Ratios of Red Cell Series to White Cell Series. In the final analysis, bone marrow cytology allows a quantitative assessment only in relative terms.

The important ratio of red precursor cells to white cells is 1 : 2 for men and 1 : 3 for women.

Shifts towards erythropoiesis are seen in all regenerative anemias (hemorrhagic anemia, iron deficiency anemia, vitamin deficiency anemia, and hemolysis), pseudopolycythemia (Gaisböck syndrome), and polycythemia, also in rare pseudo-regenerative disorders, such as sideroachrestic anemia and myelodysplasias. *Shifts toward granulopoiesis* are seen in all reactive processes (infections, tumor defense) and in all malignant processes of the white cell series (chronic myeloid leukemia, acute leukoses).

Distribution and Cell Quality in Erythropoiesis. In erythropoiesis polychromatic erythroblasts normally predominate. Proerythroblasts and basophilic erythroblasts only make up a small portion (Table **4**). Here, too, a left shift indicates an increase in immature cell types and a right shift an increase in orthochromatic erythroblasts. Qualitatively, vitamin B_{12} and folic acid deficiency lead to a typical loosening-up of the nuclear structure in proerythroblasts and to nuclear segmentation and break-up in the erythroblasts (megaloblastic erythropoiesis).

A *left shift* is seen in regenerative anemias except hemolysis. Atypical proerythroblasts predominate in megaloblastic anemia and erythremia.

A *right shift* is seen in hemolytic conditions (nests of normoblasts, erythrons).

Distribution and Cell Quality in Granulopoiesis. The same principle is valid as for erythropoiesis: the more mature the cells, the greater proportion of the series they make up. A left shift indicates a greater than normal proportion of immature cells and a right shift a greater than normal proportion of mature cells (Table **4**). Strong reactive conditions may lead to dissociations in the maturation process, e.g., the nucleus shows the structure of a myelocyte while the cytoplasm is still strongly basophilic. In malignancies, the picture is dominated by blasts, which may often be difficult to identify with any certainty.

A *left shift* is observed in all reactive processes and at the start of neoplastic transformation (smoldering anemia, refractory anemia with excess blasts [RAEB]). In acute leukemias, undifferentiated and partially matured blasts may predominate. In agranulocytosis, promyelocytes are most abundant.

A *right shift* is diagnostically irrelevant.

Cytochemistry. To distinguish between reactive processes and chronic myeloid leukemia, leukocyte alkaline phosphatase is determined in fresh smears of blood. To distinguish between different types of acute leukemia, the peroxidase and esterase reactions are carried out (pp. 97 and 99), and iron staining is performed (p. 109) if myelodysplasia is suspected.

Cytogenetic Analysis. This procedure will take the diagnosis forward in cases of leukemia and some lymphadenomas. The fresh material must be heparinized before shipment, preferably after discussion with a specialist laboratory.

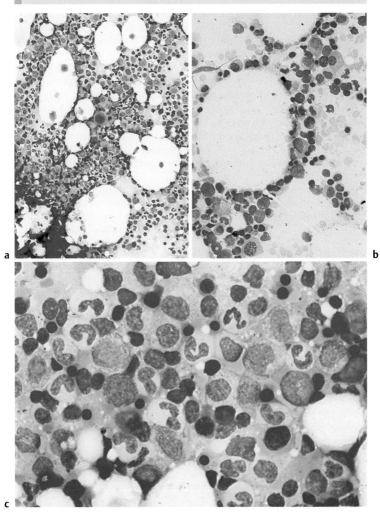

Fig. **18**   Bone marrow cytology. **a** Bone marrow cytology of normal cell density in a young adult (smear from a bone marrow spicule shown at the lower right; magnification ×100). **b** More adipocytes with large vacuoles are present in this bone marrow preparation with normal hematopoietic cell densities; usually found in older patients. **c** Normal bone marrow cytology (magnification ×400). Even this overview shows clearly that erythropoiesis (dense, black, round nuclei) accounts for only about one-third of all the cells.

Qualitative and Quantitative Assessment of the Remaining Cells. Lymphocyte counts may be slightly raised in reactive processes, but a significant increase suggests a disease of the lymphatic system. The exact classification of these disease follows the criteria of lymphocyte morphology (Fig. **16**). If elevated lymphocyte counts are found only in one preparation or within a circumscribed area, physiological lymph follicles in the bone marrow are likely to be the source. In a borderline case, the histology and analysis of lymphocyte surface markers yield more definitive data.

Plasma cell counts are also slightly elevated in reactive processes and very elevated in plasmacytoma. Reactive increase of lymphocytes and plasma cells with concomitant low counts in the other series is often an indication of panmyelopathy (aplastic anemia).

Raised *eosinophil* and *monocyte* counts in bone marrow have the same diagnostic significance as in blood (p. 44).

Megakaryocyte counts are reduced under the effects of all toxic stimuli on bone marrow. Counts increase after bleeding, in essential thrombocytopenia (Werlhof syndrome), and in myeloproliferative diseases (chronic myeloid leukemia, polycythemia, and essential thrombocythemia).

Iron Staining of Erythropoietic Cells. Perls' Prussian blue (also known as Perls' acid ferrocyanide reaction) shows the presence of ferritin in 20–40% of all normoblasts, in the form of one to four small granules. The iron-containing cells are called *sideroblasts*. Greater numbers of ferritin granules in normoblasts indicate a disorder of iron utilization (sideroachresia, especially in myelodysplasia), particularly when the granules form a ring around the nucleus (ring sideroblasts). Perls' Prussian blue reaction also stains the diffuse iron precipitates in macrophages (Fig. **19 b**).

Under exogenous iron deficiency conditions the proportion of sideroblasts and iron-storing macrophages is reduced. However, if the shift in iron utilization is due to infectious and/or toxic conditions, the iron content in normoblasts is reduced while the macrophages are loaded with iron to the point of saturation. In hemolytic conditions, the iron content of normoblasts is normal; it is elevated only in essential or symptomatic refractory anemia (including megaloblastic anemia).

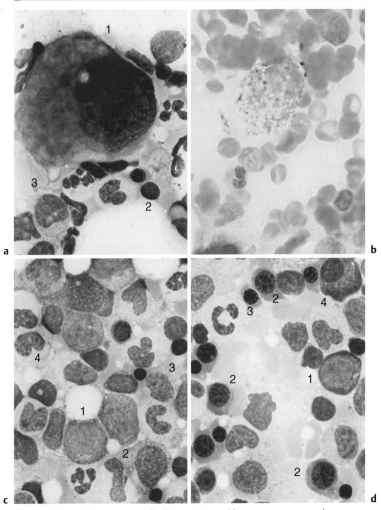

Fig. **19**　Normal bone marrow findings. **a** Normal bone marrow: megakaryocyte (1), erythroblasts (2), and myelocyte (3). **b** Iron staining in the bone marrow cytology: iron-storing macrophage. **c** Normal bone marrow with slight preponderance of granulocytopoiesis, e.g., promyelocyte (1), myelocyte (2), metamyelocyte (3), and band granulocyte (4). **d** Normal bone marrow with slight preponderance of erythropoiesis, e.g., basophilic erythroblast (1), polychromatic erythroblasts (2), and orthochromatic erythroblast (3). Compare (differential diagnosis) with the plasma cell (4) with its eccentric nucleus.

57

Bone Marrow: Medullary Stroma Cells

➤ *Fibroblastic reticular cells* form a firm but elastic matrix in which the blood-forming cells reside, and are therefore rarely found in the bone marrow aspirate or cytological smear. When present, they are most likely to appear as dense cell groups with long fiber-forming cytoplasmic processes and small nuclei. Iron staining shows them up as a group of reticular cells which, like macrophages, have the potential to store iron. If they become the prominent cell population in the bone marrow, an aplastic or toxic medullary disorder must be considered.

➤ *Reticular histiocytes* (not yet active in phagocytosis) are identical to phagocytic *macrophages* and are the main storage cells for tissue-bound iron. Because of their small nuclei and easy-flowing cytoplasm, they are noticeable after panoptic staining only when they contain obvious entities such as lipids or pigments.

➤ *Osteoblasts* are large cells with wide, eccentric nuclei. They differ from plasma cells in that the cytoplasm has no perinuclear lighter space (cell center) and stains a cloudy grayish-blue. As they are normally rare in bone marrow, increased presence of osteoblasts in the marrow may indicate metastasizing tumor cells (from another location).

➤ *Osteoclasts* are multinucleated syncytia with wide layers of grayish-blue stained cytoplasm, which often displays delicate azurophilic granulation. They are normally extremely rare in aspirates, and when they are found it is usually under the same conditions as osteoblasts. They are distinguished from megakaryocytes by their round and regular nuclei and by their lack of thrombocyte buds.

From the above, it will be seen that bone marrow findings can be assessed on the basis of a knowledge of the cells elements described above (p. 32 ff.), taking account of the eight categories given on p. 52 f. It also shows that a diagnosis from bone marrow aspirates can safely be made only in conjunction with clinical findings, blood chemistry, and the qualitative and quantitative blood values. For this reason, a table of diagnostic steps taking account of these categories is provided at the beginning of each of the following chapters.

Cells from the bone marrow stroma never occur in the blood stream

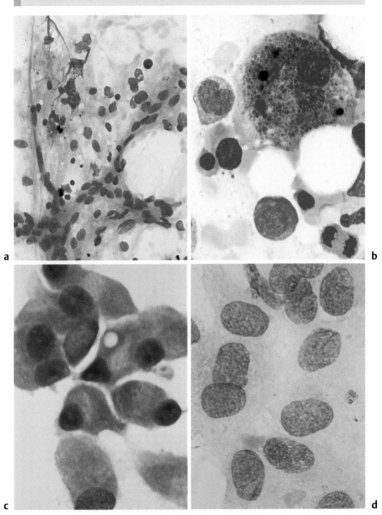

Fig. **20**   Bone marrow stroma. **a** Spindle-shaped fibroblasts form the structural framework of the bone marrow (shown here: aplastic hematopoiesis after therapy for multiple myeloma). **b** A macrophage has phagocytosed residual nuclear material (here after chemotherapy for acute leukemia). **c** Bone marrow osteoblasts are rarely found in the cytological assessment. The features that distinguish osteoblasts from plasma cells are their more loosely structured nuclei and the cloudy, "busy" basophilic cytoplasm. **d** Osteoclasts are multinucleated giant cells with wide, spreading cytoplasm.

Abnormalities of the White Cell Series

A very old-fashioned, intuitive way of classifying CBCs is to divide them into those in which round to oval (mononuclear) cells predominate and those in which segmented (polynuclear) cells predominate. However, this old method does allow the relevant differential diagnosis to be inferred from a cursory screening of a slide.

Differential Diagnostic Notes

Differential diagnosis when round to oval cells predominate

➤ Reactive lymphocytoses and monocytoses, pp. 67 f., 89
➤ Lymphatic system diseases (lymphomas, lymphocytic leukemia), p. 70
➤ Acute leukemias, including episodes of chronic myeloid leukemia (CML), p. 96 ff.
➤ Low counts of cells with segmented nuclei (agranulocytosis–aplastic anemia–myelodysplasia), pp. 86, 106, 148

Differential diagnosis when segmented cells predominate

➤ Reactive processes, p. 112 ff.
➤ Chronic myeloid leukemia, p. 114 ff.
➤ Osteomyelosclerosis, p. 122
➤ Polycythemia vera, p. 162 ff.

Predominance of Mononuclear Round to Oval Cells (Table **5**)

The cell counts (per microliter) show a wide range of values and depend on a variety of conditions even in normal blood. Any disease may therefore result in higher (leukocytosis) or lower cell counts (leukopenia). The assessment of cell counts requires the knowledge of normal values and their ranges (spreads) (Table **2**, p. 12). The most important diagnostic indicator therefore is not the cell count but the cell type. In a first assessment, mononuclear (round to oval) and polynuclear (segmented) cells are compared. This is the first step in the differential diagnosis of the multi-faceted spectrum of blood cells.

Absolute or relative predominance of mononuclear cells points to a defined set of diagnostic probabilities. The differential diagnostic notes opposite can help with a first orientation.

Consequently, the most important step is to distinguish between lymphatic cells and myeloid blasts. The nuclear morphology makes it possible to distinguish between the two cell types. In lymphatic cells the nucleus usually displays dense coarse chromatin with slate-like architecture and lighter zones between very dense ones. In contrast, the immature cells in myeloid leukemias contain nuclei with a more delicate reticular, sometimes sand-like chromatin structure with a finer, more irregular pattern.

Table 5   Diagnostic work-up for abnormalities in the white cell series with mononuclear cells predominating

Clinical findings	Hb	MCH	Leukocytes	Segmented cells	Lymphocytes (%)	Other cells
Fever, lymph nodes, possibly exanthema	n	n	↓/n	↓	↑ Stimulated forms	–
Fever, severe lymphoma, possibly spleen ↑	n	n	↑	↓	↑	Large blastic stimulated cells (DD: lymphoblasts)
Slowly progressing lymph node enlargement in several locations	↓/n	↓/n	↑	↓	↑↑	–
Night sweat, slowly progressing lymphoma (± spleen), possibly fever	↓	↓	n/↑	↓	↑	Plasmacytoid cells, possibly rouleaux formation of the erythrocytes
Slowly progressing lymph node enlargement in one or a few locations	↓	n/↓	n/↑/↓	n/↓	Possibly ↑	Possibly cells with grooves
Isolated severe splenomegaly	↓	↓	↓/↑	↓	Hairy cells	
Fever, angina	n	n	↓	↓	↑	Monocytes ↑
Diffuse general symptoms	↓	↓	↑	↓	n	Monocytes ↑
Pale skin, fever (signs of hemorrhage)	↓	↓	↑/n/↓	↓	↓	Atypical round cells predominate
Fatigue, night sweat, possibly bone pain	↓	↓	n/↓	n	n	Possibly rouleaux formations of erythrocytes

Diagnostic steps proceed from left to right. | The next step is usually unnecessary; : optional step, may not progress the diagnosis; ⟶ the next step is obligatory.

Thrombo-cytes	Electro-phoresis	Tentative diagnosis	Evidence/advanced diagnostics	Bone mar-row	Ref. page
n	n/γ↑	**Virus infection, e.g., rubeola**	Clinical developments, possibly serological tests		p. 66
n	γ↑	**Mono-nucleosis**	Mononucleosis quick test, EBV serology (cytomegaly titer?)		p. 68
n/↓	n/γ↓	**Leukemic non-Hodgkin lymphoma, esp. CLL**	Marker analysis of peripheral lymphocytes is sufficient in typical disease presentations; lymph node histology for treatment decisions, if necessary	Always involved in CLL, not always in other lymphomas	p. 74
n/↓	Possibly γ↑	**Immunocy-toma (incl. Walden-ström dis-ease)**	Immunoelectrophore-sis; marker analysis for lymphocytes in blood and bone marrow; lymph node histology in case of doubt	Usually involved	p. 78
n/↓	n	**Non-Hodgkin lymphoma, e.g. follicular lymphoma**	Lymph node histology	For the pur-pose of stag-ing, possibly positive	p. 78
↓	n	**Hairy cell leukemia**	Cell surface markers	Always involved, dis-crete in the beginning	p. 80
n	n	**Agranulo-cytosis**	⟶	Maturation arrest	p. 86
n	Possibly a₂↑	**Reactive monocytosis in chronic infection or tumor**	Determine disease origin		p. 88
↓	n	**Acute leukemia**	Cytochemistry, marker analysis, possibly cyto-genetics ⟶	Marker for blasts	p. 90 ff
n/↓	Sharp peaks ↑	**Multiple myeloma**	Immunoelectrophore-sis, skeletal X-ray ⟶	Bone marrow contains plasma cells	p. 82

Reactive Lymphocytosis

Lymphatic cells show wide variability and transform easily. This is usually seen as enlarged nuclei, a moderately loose, coarse chromatin structure, and a marked widening of the basophilic cytoplasmic layer.

Clinical findings, which include acute fever symptoms, enlarged lymph nodes, and sometimes exanthema, help to identify a lymphatic reactive state. Unlike the case in acute leukemias, erythrocyte and thrombocyte counts are not significantly reduced. Although the granulocyte count is relatively reduced, its absolute value (per microliter) rarely falls below the lower limit of normal values.

Morphologically normal lymphocytes predominate in the blood analyses in the following diseases:

➤ Whooping cough (pertussis) with clear leukocytosis and total lymphocyte counts up to 20 000 and even 50 000/μl; occasionally, slightly plasmacytoid differentiation.
➤ Infectious lymphocytosis, a pediatric infectious disease with fever of short duration. Lymphocyte counts may increase to > 50 000/μl.
➤ Chickenpox, measles, and brucellosis, in which a less well-developed relative lymphocytosis is found, and the counts remain within the normal range.
➤ Hyperthyroidism and Addison disease, which show relative lymphocytosis.
➤ Constitutional relative lymphocytosis, which can reach up to 60% and occurs without apparent reason (mostly in asthenic teenagers).
➤ Absolute granulocytopenias with relative lymphocytosis (p. 86).
➤ Chronic lymphocytic leukemia (CLL), which is always accompanied by absolute and relative lymphocytosis, usually with high cell counts.

Transformed, "stimulated" lymphocytes (*"virocytes"*) predominate in the CBC in the following diseases with reactive symptoms:

➤ *Lymphomatous toxoplasmosis* does not usually involve significant leukocytosis. Slightly plasmacytoid cell forms are found.
➤ In *rubella infections* the total leukocyte count is normal or low, and the lymphocytosis is only relatively developed. The cell morphology ranges from basophilic plasmacytoid cells to typical plasma cells.
➤ In *hepatitis* the total leukocyte and lymphocyte counts are normal. However, the lymphocytes often clearly show plasmacytoid transformation.
➤ The most extreme lymphocyte transformation is observed in *mononucleosis* (Epstein–Barr virus [EBV] or cytomegalovirus [CMV] infection) (p. 68).

During lymphatic reactive states, variable cells with dense, round nuclei (e.g., virocytes) dominate the CBC

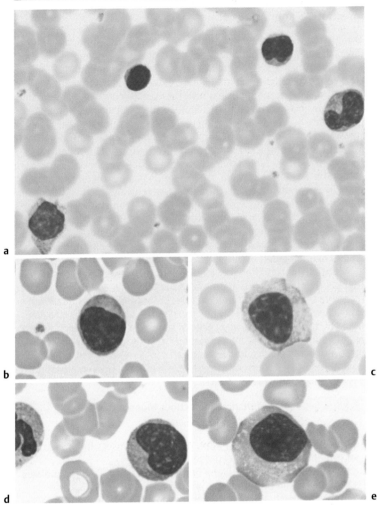

Fig. 21 Lymphatic reactive states. a–e Wide variability of the lymphatic cells in a lymphotropic infection (in this case cytomegalovirus infection). Some of the cells may resemble myelocytes, but their chromatin is always denser than myelocyte chromatin.

Examples of Extreme Lymphocytic Stimulation: Infectious Mononucleosis

Epstein–Barr virus infection should be considered when, after a prodromal fever of unknown origin, there are signs of enlarged lymph nodes and developing angina, and the blood analysis shows predominantly mononuclear cells and a slightly, or moderately, elevated leukocyte count. Varying proportions of the mononuclear cells (at least 20%) may be rather extensively transformed round cells (Pfeiffer cells, virocytes). Immunological markers are necessary to ascertain that these are stimulated lymphocytes (mostly T-lymphocytes) defending the B-lymphocyte stem population against the virus attack. The nuclei of these stimulated lymphocytes are two- to three-fold larger than those of normal lymphocytes and their chromatin has changed from a dense and coarse structure to a looser, more irregular organization. The cytoplasm is always relatively wide and more or less basophilic with vacuoles. Granules are absent. A small proportion of cells appear plasmacytoid. In the course of the disease, the degree of transformation and the proportions of the different cell morphologies change almost daily. A slight left shift and elevated monocyte count are often found in the granulocyte series.

Acute leukemia is often considered in the differential diagnosis in addition to other viral conditions, because the transformed lymphocytes can resemble the blasts found in leukemia. Absence of a quantitative reduction of hematopoiesis in all the blood cell series, however, makes leukemia unlikely, as do the variety and speed of change in the cell morphology. Finally, serological tests (EBV antigen test, test for antibodies, and, if indicated, quick tests) can add clarification.

Where serological tests are negative, the cause of the symptoms is usually cytomegalovirus rather than EBV.

Characteristics of Infectious Mononucleosis

Age of onset: School age
Clinical findings: Enlarged lymph nodes (rapid onset), inflammations of throat and possibly spleen ↑
CBC: Leukocytes ↑, stimulated lymph nodes, partially lymphoblasts (hematocrit and thrombocytes are normal)
Further diagnostics: EBV serological test (IgM +), transaminases usually ↑
Differential diagnosis: Lymphomas (usually without fever), leukemia (usually Hb ↓, thrombocytes ↓) Persistent disease (more than 3 weeks): possibly test for blood cell markers, lymph node cytology (→ histology)
Course, treatment: Spontaneous recovery within 2–4 weeks; general palliation

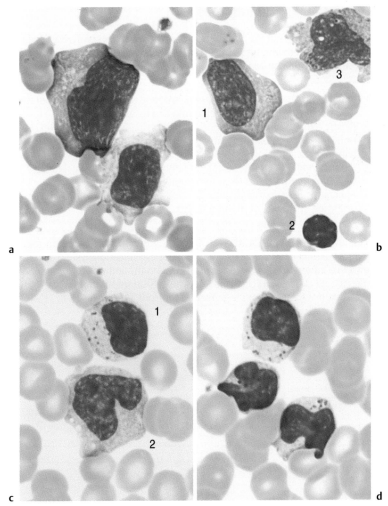

Fig. **22** Lymphocytes during viral infection. **a** "Blastic," lymphatic reactive form (Pfeiffer cell), in addition to less reactive virocytes in Epstein–Barr virus (EBV) infection. This phase with blastic cells lasts only a few days. **b** Virocyte (1) with homogeneous deep blue stained cytoplasm in EBV infection, in addition to normal lymphocyte (2) and monocyte (3). **c** Virus infection can also lead to elevated counts of large granulated lymphocytes (LGL) (1). Monocyte (2). **d** Severe lymphatic stress reaction with granulated lymphocytes. A lymphoma must be considered if this finding persists.

Diseases of the Lymphatic System (Non-Hodgkin Lymphomas)

Malignant diseases of the lymphatic system are further classified as Hodgkin and non-Hodgkin lymphomas (NHL). NHL will be discussed here because most NHLs can be diagnosed on the blood analysis.

➤ *Non-Hodgkin lymphomas* arise mostly from small or blastic B-cells.
➤ Small-cell NHL cells are usually leukemic and relatively indolent, of the type of chronic lymphocytic leukemia and its variants.
➤ *Blastic NHL* (precursor lymphoma) is not usually leukemic. An exception is the lymphoblastic lymphoma, which takes its course as an acute lymphocytic leukemia.
➤ *Plasmacytoma* is an osteotropic B-cell lymphoma that releases not its cells but their products (immunoglobulins) into the bloodstream.
➤ *Malignant lymphogranulomatosis* (Hodgkin disease) cannot be diagnosed on the basis of blood analysis. It is therefore discussed under lymph node cytology (p. 176).

The modern pathological classification of lymphomas is based on morphology and cell immunology. The updated classification system according to Lennert (Kiel) has been adopted in Germany and was recently modified to reflect the WHO classification. The definitions of stages I–IV in NHL agree with the Ann Arbor classification for Hodgkin's disease.

Table **6 a**   Classification of non-Hodgkin: comparison of the relevant classes in the Kiel and WHO classifications

WHO	Kiel	Clinical Characteristics	Marker*
Precursor lymphomas/leukemias			
➤ Precursor-B-lymphoblastic lymphoma	B-lymphoblastic lymphoma	Aggressive	Tdt, CD19, 22, 79 a
➤ Precursor B-cell active lymphoblastic leukemia	B-ALL		
Mature B-cell lymphoma			
➤ Chronic lymphocytic leukemia	B-CLL	Usually indolent	CD5, 19, 20, 23 tris 12 or 13q-, 11q-, 6q-, p53
– contains the lymphoplasmacytoid immunocytoma	Lymphoplasmacytoid immunocytoma	Usually indolent	
➤ B-cell prolymphocytic leukemia		Aggressive	

Table **6a**   Continued

WHO	Kiel	Clinical Characteristics	Marker*
➤ Lymphoplasmacytic leukemia	Lymphoplasmacytic immunocytoma	Sometimes IgM paraprotein (Waldenström disease)	–/+ CD5
➤ Mantle cell lymphoma	Centrocytic lymphoma	Usually aggressive	– CD23, CD5 t(11;14) bcl-1 rearr.
➤ Marginal zone lymphoma		Usually aggressive	–CD5, CD23
– Nodal	Monocytoid lymphoma	sive	
– Extranodal in mucosa (MALT)	MALT (mucosa-assoc. lymphoid tissue) lymphoma	Often indolent	
– Lienal (splenic)	Lymphoma with splenomegaly		
➤ Follicular lymphoma	Centroblastic/centro-cytic lymphoma;	Usually indolent	–CD5, ± CD10
– Grade 1, 2			t(14;18)
– Grade 3 (a, b)	centroblastic lymphoma (a), secondary (b), follic-ular	Highly malignant	bcl2
➤ Hairy cell leukemia	Hairy cell leukemia	Usually indolent	–CD103, CD11c, CD25 t(2;8) t(8;14)
➤ Plasma cell myeloma (plasma-cytoma)	[Plasmacytoma is not included in the Kiel classification]		CD 138
– Monoclonal hypergamma-globulinemia (GUS)			
– Solitary bone plasmacytoma			
– Extraosseous bone plasmacy-toma			
– Primary amyloidosis			
– Heavy-chain disease			
Primary large-cell lymphoma			
➤ Diffuse large-cell B-cell lymphoma	Centroblastic Immunoblastic	Extremely malig-nant	CD20, 79a, 19, 22
– Centroblastic	Large-cell anaplastic	Extremely malig-nant	
– Immunoblastic			
– Large-cell anaplastic		Extremely malig-nant	
➤ Burkitt lymphoma	Burkitt lymphoma	Extremely malig-nant	t(2;8) t(8;14) myc

* Cited markers are positive, absent markers are indicated with a minus sign.

Table **6 b**   T-cell lymphomas (since T-cell lymphomas make up only 10 % of all NHLs, this table gives just a brief characterization; for markers see Table **7**)

WHO (≈ Kiel)		Clinical characteristics
Classification	Manifestation	
➤ T-prolymphocytic leukemia	Leukemic	Aggressive
➤ Large granular lymphocyte leukemia (LGL)	Leukemic	Sometimes indolent
➤ T-cell lymphoblastic leukemia	Leukemic	Aggressive
➤ Sézary syndrome, mycosis fungoides	Cutaneous	Chronic, progressive
➤ Angioimmunoblastic T-cell lymphoma (AILD)	Nodal and ENT	Usually aggressive
➤ Lymphoblastic T-cell lymphoma	Nodal	Aggressive
➤ T-cell zone lymphoma (nonspecific peripheral lymphoma)	Nodal	Sometimes slowly progressive
➤ Lennert lymphoma with multifocal epithelioid cells	Nodal	Sometimes slowly progressive
➤ Large-cell anaplastic lymphoma (ki1)	Nodal	Aggressive

Differentiation of the Lymphatic Cells and Cell Surface Marker Expression in Non-Hodgkin Lymphoma Cells

Non-Hodgkin lymphoma cells derive monoclonally from specific stages in the B- or T-cell differentiation, and their surface markers reflect this. The surface markers are identified in immunocytological tests (Table **7**) carried out on heparinized blood or bone marrow spicules.

The blastic lymphomas will not be discussed further in the context of diagnostics based on blood cell morphology. The findings in the primarily leukemic forms of the disease, such as lymphoblastic lymphoma, resemble those for ALL (p. 104). Other blastic lymphomas can usually only be diagnosed on the basis of lymph node tissue (Fig. **65**). Of course, despite all the progress in the analysis of blood cell differentiation, often analysis of histological slides in conjunction with the blood analysis is required for a confident diagnosis.

Table 7   Cell surface markers of lymphatic cells in leukemic, low-grade malignant non-Hodgkin lymphoma

Marker	B-CLL	B-PLL	HCL	FL	MCL	SLVL	T-CLL	GL	SS	T-PLL	ATLL
S Ig	(+)	++	++	++	++	++	–	–	–	–	–
CD 2	–	–	–	–	–	–	+	+	+	+	+
CD 3	–	–	–	–	–	–	+	–	+	+	+
CD 4	–	–	–	–	–	–	–	–	+	+/–	+
CD 5	++	–	–	–	+	–	–	–	+	+	+
CD 7	–	–	–	–	–	–	–	–	+/–	+	–/+
CD 8	–	–	–	–	–	–	+	+/–	+/–	+/–	+/–
CD 19/20/24	++	++	++	+	+	++	–	–	–	–	–
CD 22	+/–	++	++	+	+	++	–	–	–	–	–
CD 10	–	–	–	+/–	–	–	–	–	–	–	–
CD 25	–	–	++	–	–	+/–	+	–	–	–	+
CD 56	–	–	–	–	–	–	–	+	–	–	–
CD 103	–	–	++	–	–	–	–	–	–	–	–

CLL chronic lymphocytic leukemia; PLL prolymphocytic leukemia; HCL hairy cell leukemia; FL follicular lymphoma; MCL mantle cell lymphoma; SLVL splenic lymphoma with villous lymphocytes; LGL large granular lymphocyte leukemia; SS Sézary syndrome; ATLL adult T-cell lymphoma.

Chronic Lymphocytic Leukemia (CLL) and Related Diseases

A chronic lymphadenoma, or chronic lymphocytic leukemia, can sometimes be clinically diagnosed with some certainty. An example is the case of a patient (usually older) with clearly enlarged lymph nodes and significant lymphocytosis (in 60% of the cases this is greater than 20 000/μl and in 20% of the cases it is greater than 100 000/μl) in the absence of symptoms that point to a reactive disorder. The lymphoma cells are relatively small, and the nuclear chromatin is coarse and dense. The narrow layer of slightly basophilic cytoplasm does not contain granules. Shadows around the nucleus are an artifact produced by chromatin fragmentation during preparation (Gumprecht's nuclear shadow). In order to confirm the diagnosis, the B-cell markers on circulating lymphocytes should be characterized to show that the cells are indeed monoclonal. The transformed lymphocytes are dispersed at varying cell densities throughout the bone marrow and the lymph nodes. A slowly progressing hypogammaglobulinemia is another important indicator of a B-cell maturation disorder.

Transition to a diffuse large-cell B-lymphoma (Richter syndrome) is rare: B-prolymphocytic leukemia (B-PLL) displays unique symptoms. At least 55% of the lymphocytes in circulating blood have large central vacuoles. When 15–55% of the cells are prolymphocytes, the diagnosis of atypical CLL, or transitional CLL/PLL is confirmed. In some CLL-like diseases, the layer of cytoplasm is slightly wider. B-CLL was defined as *lymphoplasmacytoid immunocytoma* in the Kiel classification. According to the WHO classification, it is a B-CLL variation (compare this with lymphoplasmacytic leukemia, p. 78). CLL of the T-lymphocytes is rare. The cells show nuclei with either invaginations or well-defined nucleoli (*T-prolymphocytic leukemia*). The leukemic phase of cutaneous T-cell lymphoma (CTCL) is known as Sézary syndrome. The cell elements in this syndrome and T-PLL are similar.

Fig. **23**   CLL. **a** Extensive proliferation of lymphocytes with densely structured ▶ nuclei and little variation in CLL. Nuclear shadows are frequently seen, a sign of the fragility of the cells (magnification ×400). **b** Lymphocytes in CLL with typical coarse chromatin structure and small cytoplasmic layer (enlargement of a section from 23 **a,** magnification ×1000); only discreet nucleoli may occur. **c** Slightly eccentric enlargement of the cytoplasm in the lymphoplasmacytoid variant of CLL.

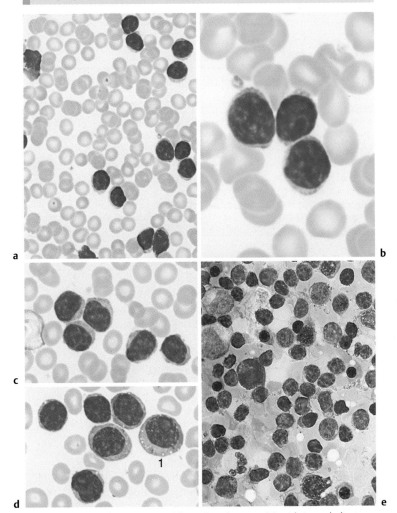

Fig. **23** **d** Proliferation of atypical large lymphocytes (1) with irregularly structured nucleus, well-defined nucleolus, and wide cytoplasm (atypical CLL or transitional form CLL/PLL). **e** Bone marrow cytology in CLL: There is always strong proliferation of the typical small lymphocytes, which are usually spread out diffusely.

Table **8** Staging of CLL according to Rai (1975)

Stage		Identifying criteria/definition
(Low risk)	**0**	Lymphocytosis > 15 000/µl Bone marrow infiltration > 40 %
(Intermediate risk)	**I**	Lymphocytosis and lymphadenopathy
	II	Lymphocytosis and hepatomegaly and/or spleno-megaly (with or without lymphadenopathy)
(High risk)	**III**	Lymphocytosis and anemia (Hb < 11.0 g/dl) (with or without lymphadenopathy and/or organomegaly)
	IV	Lymphocytosis and thrombopenia (< 100 000/µl) (with or without anemia, lymphadenopathy, or organomegaly)

Table **9** Staging of CLL according to Binet (1981)

Stage	Identifying criteria/definition
A	Hb > 10.0 g/dl, normal thrombocyte count < 3 regions with enlarged lymph nodes
B	Hb > 10.0 g/dl, normal thrombocyte count > 3 regions with enlarged lymph nodes
C	Hb < 10.0 g/dl and/or thrombocyte count < 100 000/µl independent of the number of affected locations

Characteristics of CLL

Age of onset: Mature adulthood

Clinical presentation: Gradual enlargement of all lymph nodes, usu-ally moderately enlarged spleen, slow onset of anemia and increasing susceptibility to infections, later thrombocytopenia

CBC: In all cases absolute lymphocytosis; in the course of the disease Hb ↓, thrombocytes ↓, immunoglobulin ↓

Further diagnostics: Lymphocyte surface markers (see pp. 68 ff.); bone marrow (always infiltrated); lymph node histology further clarifies the diagnosis

Differential diagnosis: (a) Related lymphomas: marker analysis, lymph node histology; (b) acute leukemia: cell surface marker analy-sis, cytochemistry, cytogenetics (pp. 88 ff.)

Course, therapy: Individually varying, usually fairly indolent course; in advanced stages or fast progressing disease: moderate chemother-apy (cell surface marker, see Table **7**)

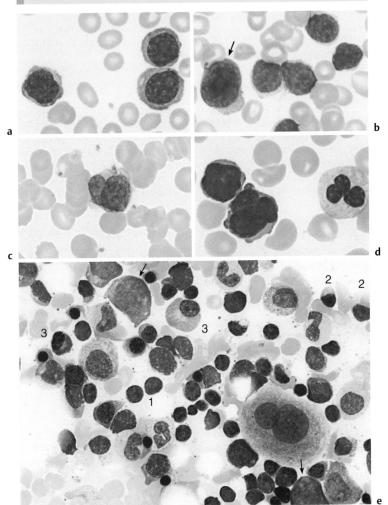

Fig. **24** Lymphoma of the B-cell and T-cell lineages. **a** Prevalence of large lymphocytes with clearly defined nucleoli and wide cytoplasm: prolymphocytic leukemia of the B-cell series (B-PLL). **b** The presence of large blastic cells (arrow) in CLL suggest a rare transformation (Richter syndrome). **c** The rare Sézary syndrome (T-cell lymphoma of the skin) is characterized by irregular, indented lymphocytes. **d** Prolymphocytic leukemia of the T-cell series (T-PLL) with indented nuclei and nucleoli (rare). **e** Bone marrow in lymphoplasmacytic immunocytoma: focal or diffuse lymphocyte infiltration (e.g., 1), plasmacytoid lymphocytes (e.g., 2) and plasma cells (e.g., 3). Red cell precursors predominate (e.g., basophilic erythroblasts, arrow).

The pathological staging for CLL is always Ann Arbor stage IV because the bone marrow is affected. In the classifications of disease activity by Rai and Binet (analogous to that for leukemic immunocytoma), the transition between stages is smooth (Tables **8** and **9**).

Lymphoplasmacytic Lymphoma

The CBC shows lymphocytes with relatively wide layers of cytoplasm. The bone marrow contains a mixture of lymphocytes, plasmacytic lymphocytes, and plasma cells. In up to 30% of cases paraprotein is secreted, predominantly monoclonal IgM. This constitutes the classic Waldenström syndrome (Waldenström macroglobulinemia). The differential diagnosis may call for exclusion of the rare plasma cell leukemia (see p. 82) and of lymphoplasmacytoid immunocytoma, which is closely related to CLL (see p. 74).

Characteristics

➤ *Lymphoplasmacytoid immunocytoma:* This is a special form of B-CLL in which usually only a few precursors migrate into the bloodstream (a lesser degree of malignancy). A diagnosis may only be possible on the basis of bone marrow or lymph node analysis.

➤ *Lymphoplasmacytic lymphoma:* Few precursors migrate into the bloodstream (i.e., bone marrow or lymph node analysis is sometimes necessary). There is often secretion of IgM paraprotein, which can lead to hyperviscosity.

Further diagnostics: Marker analyses in circulating cells, lymph node cytology, bone marrow cytology and histology, and immunoelectrophoresis. Plasmacytoma cells migrate into the circulating blood in appreciable numbers in only 1–2% of all cases of plasma cell leukemia. Therefore, paraproteins must be analyzed in bone marrow aspirates (p. 82).

Facultative Leukemic Lymphomas
(e.g., Mantle Cell Lymphoma and Follicular Lymphoma)

In all cases of non-Hodgkin lymphoma, the transformed cells may migrate into the blood stream. This is usually observed in *mantle cell lymphoma*: The cells are typically of medium size. On close examination, their nuclei show loosely structured chromatin and they are lobed with small indentations (cleaved cells). Either initially, or, more commonly, during the course of the disease, a portion of cells becomes larger with relatively enlarged nuclei (diameter 8–12 μm). These larger cells are variably "blastoid." Lymphoid cells also migrate into the blood in stage IV *follicular lymphoma*.

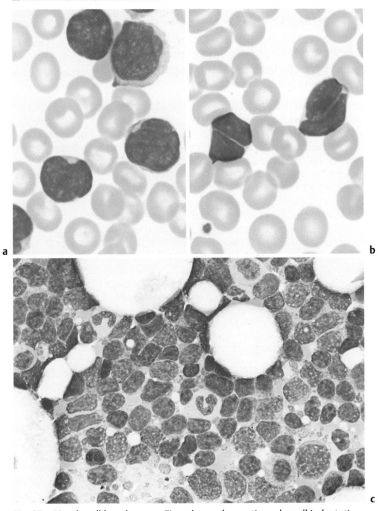

Fig. **25** Mantle cell lymphoma. **a** Fine, dense chromatin and small indentations of the nuclei suggest migration of leukemic mantle cell lymphoma cells into the blood stream. **b** Denser chromatin and sharp indentations suggest migration of follicular lymphoma cells into the blood stream. **c** Diffuse infiltration of the bone marrow with polygonal, in some cases indented lymphatic cells in mantle cell lymphoma. Bone marrow involvement in follicular lymphoma can often only be demonstrated by histological and cytogenetic studies.

"Monocytoid" cells with a wide layer of only faintly staining cytoplasm occur in blood in *marginal zone lymphadenoma* (differential diagnosis: lymphoplasmacytic immunocytoma).

Lymphoma, Usually with Splenomegaly (e.g., Hairy Cell Leukemia and Splenic Lymphoma with Villous Lymphocytes)

Hairy cell leukemia (HCL). In cases of slowly progressive general malaise with isolated splenomegaly and pancytopenia revealed by CBC (leukocytopenia, anemia, and thrombocytopenia), the *predominating mononuclear cells* deserve particular attention. The nucleus is oval, often kidney bean-shaped, and shows a delicate, elaborate chromatin structure. The cytoplasm is basophilic and stains slightly gray. Long, very thin cytoplasmic processes give the cells the hairy appearance that gave rise to the term "hairy cell leukemia" used in the international literature. The disease affects the spleen, liver, and bone marrow. Severe lymphoma is usually absent. Aside from the typical hairy cells with their long, thin processes, there are also cells with a smooth plasma membrane, similar to cells in immunocytoma. A variant shows well-defined nucleoli (HCL-V, hairy cell leukemia variant). A bone marrow aspirate often does not yield material for an analysis ("punctio sicca" or "empty tap") because the marrow is very fibrous. Apart from the bone marrow histology, *advanced cell diagnostics* are therefore very important, in particular in the determination of blood cell surface markers (immunophenotyping). This analysis reveals CD 103 and 11 c as specific markers and has largely replaced the test for tartrate-resistant acid phosphatase.

Splenic lymphoma with villous lymphocytes (SLVL). This lymphatic system disease mostly affects the spleen. There is little involvement of the bone marrow and no involvement of the lymph nodes. The blood contains lymphatic cells, which resemble hairy cells. However, the "hairs," i.e., cytoplasmic processes, are thicker and mostly restricted to one area at the cell pole, and the CD 103 marker is absent.

> **!** Splenomegaly may develop in all non-Hodgkin lymphomas. In hairy cell leukemia, the rare splenic lymphadenoma with villous lymphocytes (SLVL) and marginal zone lymphadenoma may be seen. These mostly affect the spleen.

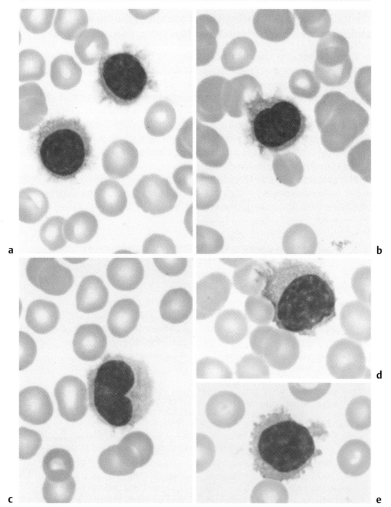

Fig. 26 Hairy cell leukemia and splenic lymphoma. **a** and **b** Ovaloid nuclei and finely "fraying" cytoplasm are characteristics of cells in hairy cell leukemia (HCL). **c** Occasionally, the hairy cell processes appear merely fuzzy. **d** and **e** When the cytoplasmic processes look thicker and much less like hair, diagnosis of the rare splenic lymphoma with villous lymphocytes (SLVL) must be considered. Here, too, the next diagnostic step is analysis of cell surface markers.

Monoclonal Gammopathy (Hypergammaglobulinemia), Multiple Myeloma*, Plasma Cell Myeloma, Plasmacytoma

Plasmacytoma is the result of malignant transformation of the most mature B-lymphocytes (Fig. **1**, p. 2). For this reason the diagnostics of this disease will be discussed here, even though migration of its specific cells into the blood stream (plasma cell leukemia) is extremely rare (1–2%).

Immunoelectrophoresis of serum and urine is performed when electrophoresis shows very discrete gammaglobulin, or globulin, fractions, or when hypogammaglobulinemia is found (in light-chain plasmacytoma). A wide range of possibilities arises for the differential diagnosis of monoclonal transformed cells (Table **10**).

The presence of more than 10% of plasma cells, or atypical plasma cells in the bone marrow, is an important diagnostic factor in the diagnosis of plasmacytoma. For more criteria, see p. 84.

Table **10**   Differential diagnosis of monoclonal hypergammaglobulinemia

Type	Characteristics
Benign disorders	
➤ Essential hypergammaglobuline-mia = MGUS (monoclonal gammopathy of unknown significance)	Usually in advanced age < 10%, plasma cells found in the bone marrow, no progression, normal polyclonal Ig
➤ Symptomatic hypergammaglobulinemia, secondary to – Infections – Tumors – Autoimmune disease	All ages (otherwise as above)
Malignant diseases	
➤ Plasmocytoma (usually IgG, A or light-chain [Bence Jones protein], rarely IgM, D, E) 90% disseminated (multiple myeloma), 5% solitary, 5% extramedullary (like a lymphoma or ENT tumor)	– Osteolysis or X-ray with severe osteoporosis – Plasmocytosis of the bone marrow > 10% – Monoclonal gammaglobulin in serum/urine with progression
➤ Lymphoma e. g., immunocytoma, CLL (potentially all lymphomas of the B-cell series)	– Enlarged lymph nodes – Usually blood lymphocytosis – Monoclonal immunoglobulin, usually IgM

* The current WHO classification suggests "multiple myeloma" (MM) for generalized plasmacytoma and "plasmacytoma" only for the rare solitary or nonosseous form of plasmacytoma.

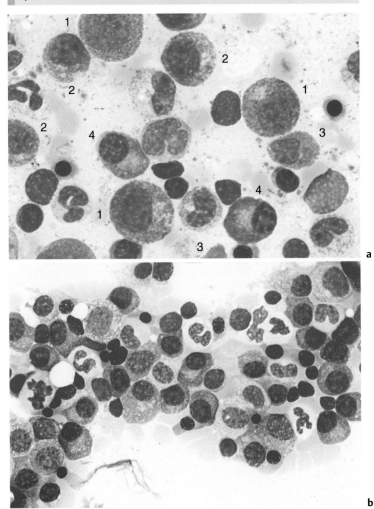

Fig. 27 Reactive plasmacytosis and plasmacytoma. **a** Bone marrow cytology with clear reactive features in the granulocyte series: strong granulation of promyelocytes (1) and myelocytes (2), eosinophilia (3), and plasma cell proliferation (4): reactive plasmacytosis (magnification ×630). **b** Extensive (about 50%) infiltration of the bone marrow of mostly well-differentiated plasma cells: multiple myeloma (magnification × 400).

Variability of Plasmacytoma Morphology

It is not easy to visually distinguish malignant cells from normal plasma cells. Like lymphocytes, normal plasma cells have a densely structured nucleus. Plasma cell nuclei with radial chromatin organization, known as "wheel-spoke nuclei," are mostly seen during histological analysis.

The following attributes suggest a malignant character of plasma cells: the cells are unusually large (Fig. **28 c**), they contain crystalline inclusions or protein inclusions ("Russell bodies") (Fig. **28 b**), or they have more than one nucleus (Fig. **28 c**).

In the differential diagnosis, they must be distinguished from hematopoietic precursor cells (Fig. **28 d**), osteoblasts (Fig. **20 c**), and blasts in acute leukemias (see Fig. **31**, p. 97).

Bone marrow involvement may be focal or in rare cases even solitary. Aside from cytological tests, bone marrow histology assays are therefore indicated. Sometimes, the biopsy must be obtained from a clearly identified osteolytic region.

Although plasmacytomas progress *slowly*, staging criteria are available (staging according to Salmon and Durie) (Table **11**).

Therapy may be put on hold in stage I. Smoldering indolent myeloma can be left for a considerable time without the introduction of therapy stress. However, chemotherapy is indicated once the myeloma has exceeded the stage 1 criteria.

Table **11**   Staging of plasmacytomas according to Salmon and Durie

Stage I	Stage II
All the following are present:	Findings fulfill neither stage I nor stage III criteria
– Hb > 10 g/dl	
– Serum calcium is normal	**Stage III**
– X-ray shows normal bone structure or solitary skeletal plasmacytoma	One or more of the following are present:
– IgG < 5 g/dl* IgA < 3 g/dl* Light chains in the urine* < 4 g/24 h	– Hb < 8.5 g/dl
	– Serum calcium is elevated
	– X-ray shows advanced bone lesions
	– IgG > 7 g/dl* IgA > 5 g/dl* Light chains in the urine: > 12 g/24 h

* Monoclonal in each case.

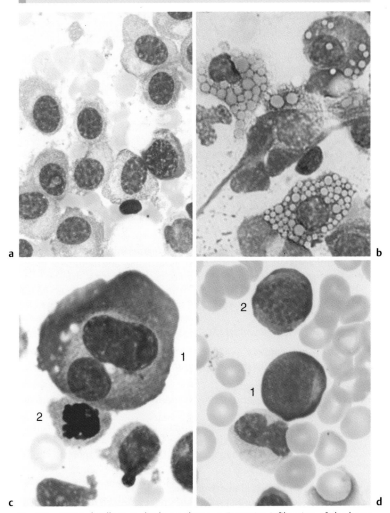

Fig. 28 Atypical cells in multiple myeloma. **a** Extensive infiltration of the bone marrow by loosely structured, slightly dedifferentiated plasma cells with wide cytoplasm in multiple myeloma. **b** In multiple myeloma, vacuolated cytoplasmic protein precipitates (Russell bodies) may be seen in plasma cells but are without diagnostic significance. **c** Binuclear plasma cells are frequently observed in multiple myeloma (1). Mitotic red cell precursor (2). **d** Differential diagnosis: red cell precursor cells can sometimes look like plasma cells. Proerythroblast (1) and basophilic erythroblast (2).

Relative Lymphocytosis Associated with Granulocytopenia (Neutropenia) and Agranulocytosis

Neutropenia is defined by a decrease in the number of neutrophilic granulocytes with segmented nuclei to less than 1500/μl (1.5×10^9/l). A neutrophil count of less than 500/μl (0.5×10^9/l) constitutes agranulocytosis. Absolute granulocytopenias with benign cause develop into relative lymphocytoses.

In the most common clinical picture, drug-induced acute agranulocytosis, the bone marrow is either poor in cells or lacks granulopoietic precursor cells (aplastic state), or shows a "maturation block" at the myeloblast–promyelocyte stage. The differential diagnosis of pure agranulocytosis versus aplasias of several cell lines is outlined on page 146.

Classification of Neutropenias and Agranulocytoses

1. Drug-induced:
   a) Dose-independent—*acute agranulocytosis.* Caused by hypersensitivity reactions: for example to pyrazolone, antirheumatic drugs (anti-inflammatory agents), antibiotics, or thyrostatic drugs.
   b) Relatively dose-dependent—*subacute agranulocytosis* (observed for carbamazepine [Tegretol], e.g. antidepressants, and cytostatic drugs).
   c) Dose-dependent—cytostatic drugs, immunosuppressants.

2. Infection-induced:
   a) E.g., EBV, hepatitis, typhus, brucellosis.

3. Autoimmune neutropenia:
   a) With antibody determination of T-cell or NK-cell autoimmune response
   b) In cases of systemic lupus erythematosus (SLE), *Pneumocystis carinii* pneumonia (PCP), Felty syndrome
   c) In cases of selective hypoplasia of the granulocytopoiesis ("pure white cell aplasia")

4. Congenital and familial neutropenias:
   Various pediatric forms; sometimes not expressed until adulthood, e.g. cyclical neutropenia

5. Secondary neutropenia in bone marrow disease:
   Myelodysplastic syndromes (MDS), e.g., acute leukemia, plasmacytoma, pernicious anemia

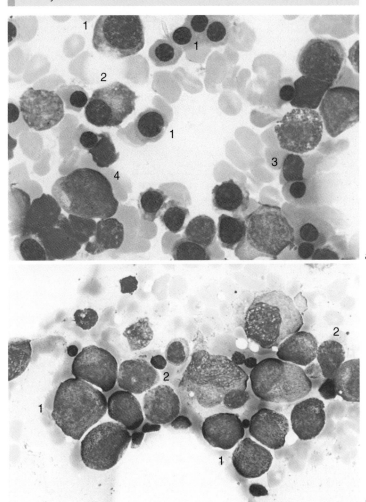

Fig. **29** The bone marrow in agranulocytosis. **a** In the early phase of agranulocytosis the bone marrow shows only red cell precursor cells (e.g., 1), plasma cells (2), and lymphocytes (3); in this sample a myeloblast—a sign of regeneration—is already present (4). **b** Bone marrow in agranulocytosis during the promyelocytic phase, showing almost exclusively promyelocytes (e.g., 1); increased eosinophilic granulocytes (2) are also present.

Monocytosis

If mononuclear cells stand out in showing an unusually elaborate nuclear structure with ridges and lobes and a wider cytoplasmic layer with very delicate granules (for characteristics see p. 46, for cell function, see p. 6), and this is in the context of relative ($> 10\%$) or absolute monocytosis (cell count $> 900/\mu l$), a series of possible triggers must be considered (Table **12**). If the morphology does not clearly identify the cells as monocytes, then esterase assays should be done in a hematological laboratory using unstained smears.

Table **12**   Possible causes of monocytosis

Infection	**Chronic reactive condition** of the immune system, e. g., in:
Nonspecific monocytosis occurs in many bacterial infections during recuperation from or in the chronic phase of:	– Autoimmune diseases
	– Chronic dermatoses
	– Regional ileitis
– Mononucleosis (aside from stimulated lymphocytes there are also monocytes)	– Sarcoidosis
	Paraneoplasm
– Listeriosis	(as attempted immune defense), e. g., in:
– Acute viral hepatitis	
– Parotitis epidemica (mumps)	– Large solid tumors
– Chickenpox	– Lymphogranulomatosis
– Recurrent fever	
– Syphilis	**Neoplasm**
– Tuberculosis	– Chronic myelomonocytic leukemia (CMML, p. 107)
– Endocarditis lenta	
– Brucellosis (Bang disease)	– Acute monocytic leukemia (p. 100)
– Variola vera (smallpox)	
– Rocky mountain spotted fever	– Acute myelomonocytic leukemia (p. 98)
– Malaria	
– Paratyphoid fever	
– Kala-azar	
– Thypus fever	
– Trypanosomiasis (African sleeping sickness)	

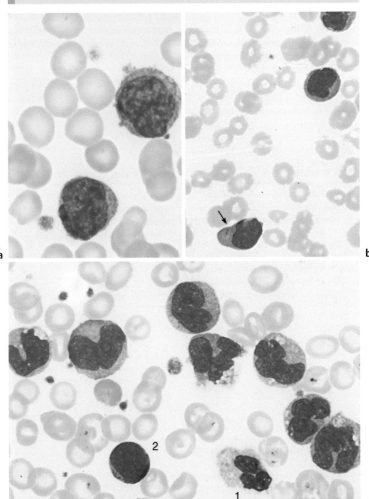

Fig. **30**   Reactive monocytosis and monocytic leukemia. **a** Reactive and neoplastic monocytes are morphologically indistinguishable; here two relatively condensed monocytes in reactive monocytosis are shown. **b** Whenever monocytes are found exclusively, a malignant etiology is likely: in this case AML M$_{5b}$ according to the FAB classification (see p. 100). Auer bodies (arrow). **c** Monocytes of different degrees of maturity, segmented neutrophilic granulocytes (1), and a small myeloblast (2) in chronic myelomonocytic leukemia (CMML, see p. 107).

Acute Leukemias

Acute leukemias are described in this place for morphological reasons, because they involve a predominance of mononuclear cells (p. 63). Although—or perhaps because—the term "leukemia" is relatively imprecise, an overview seems required (Table **13**).

The cellular phenomenon common to the different forms of leukemia is the rapidly progressive reduction in numbers of mature granulocytes, thrombocytes, and erythrocytes. Simultaneously, the leukocyte count usually increases due to the occurrence of atypical round cells.

Table **13**   Overview of all forms of leukemia

Type of leukemia	Classification/clinical findings
Acute leukemias (AL→AML, ALL)	
– Myeloid M$_{0-7}$ (incl. monocytic, erythroid, megakaryoblastic leukemias)	Always acute disease, often with fever and tendency to hemorrhage
– Lymphocytic	There may be lymphoma and thymus infiltrates
Chronic myeloid leukemia (CML)	
– Persistent leukemic diseases of the myeloproliferative system (p. 114)	Chronic disease, usually with splenomegaly
Chronic lymphocytic leukemia (CLL) and other leukemic lymphomas	
– B-CLL (90%), T-CLL (p.74 f.)	– Chronic lymphocytic leukemia,
– Prolymphocytic leukemia (p.77)	(rarely) prolymphocytic
– Hairy cell leukemia (p.80)	leukemia and hairy cell leukemia are primary leukemic lymphomas with a chronic course. All other non-Hodgkin lymphomas can develop secondary leukemic disease
Chronic myelomonocytic leukemia (CMML)	
– Leukemic form of myelodysplasia (p.106) is classified between myelodysplasia and myeloproliferative diseases	Subacute disease with transitions into acute forms of myeloid leukemia (secondary AML following MDS)

> Note that in about one-fourth of all leukemias total leukocyte counts are normal, or even reduced, and the atypical round cells affect only the relative (differential) blood analysis ("aleukemic leukemia").

In all forms of leukemia, the more fluffy layered areas of a smear show that the nuclear chromatin structure is not dense and coarse, as in a normal lymphocyte nucleus (p. 49), but more delicately structured and irregular, often "sand-like". A careful blood cell analysis should be carried out—perhaps with the assistance of a specialist laboratory—before bone marrow analysis is performed.

In most cases, the high leukocyte count facilitates the diagnosis of leukemia. Apart from the leukemia-specific blast cells, a variable number of segmented neutrophilic granulocytes may also remain, depending on the disease progression at the time of diagnosis. This gap in the cell series between blasts and mature cells is called "leukemic hiatus." It is found in ALL but not in reactive responses or chronic myeloid leukemia, which show a continuous left shift. Morphological or differential diagnosis of acute leukemia is followed by the diagnostic work-up that continues with *cytochemical tests. Immunological identification* of leukemia cells is always indicated (Table **14**).

> Diagnostic work-up when acute leukemia is suspected:
> CBC, cytochemistry, bone marrow. Collection of material to identify cell surface markers, cytogenetics, molecular genetics.

Morphological and Cytochemical Cell Identification

After a first-line diagnosis of acute leukemia has been arrived at on the basis of the cell morphology (see above), the diagnosis must be refined by cytochemical testing of blood cells or bone marrow (on fresh smears). Table **14** shows a leukemia classification based on both morphological and cytochemical criteria. The table shows that a peroxidase test allows leukemias to be classified as *peroxidase-positive* (myeloid or monocytic) or *peroxidase-negative* (lymphoblastic). The next step is the immunological classification based on cell markers.

In routine clinical hematology, the FAB classification (Table **14**) will be with us for a few more years.

Table **14**   Classification of the acute nonlymphatic leukemias by morphology, cytochemistry, and immunology

FAB type*		Peroxidase	PAS	α-Naph-thyl-acetat-esterase	Naph-thyl-ASD-esterase	Immuno-phenotype
M_0	AML with minimal marker differentia-tion, undifferen-tiated blasts without granules; distinguished from M_1 and ALL only by immunopheno-typing	< 3%	∅	∅	∅	CD 13 ⊕ or CD 33 ⊕ or MPO ⊕ CD 79a ⊖ and cyCD 3 ⊖ and cyCD 22 ⊖ and CD 61/ CD 41 ⊖ and CD 14 ⊖
M_1	AML with distinct marker differentiation (but without morpho-logical differentia-tion); sporadic dis-crete cytoplasmic granulation possible	≥ 3%	Negative to fine gran.	∅	∅	MPO ⊕ and CD 13/CD 33/ CD 65s ⊕/⊖ and CD 14 ⊖
M_2	AML with morpho-logically mature cells; > 10% of the blasts contain very small granules	> 3%	Negative to fine gran.	∅	∅	MPO ⊕ and CD 13/CD 33/ CD 65s/ CD 15 ⊕/⊖ and CD 14 ⊖
M_3	Acute promyelo-cytic leukemia; the predominant pro-myelocytes contain copious granules, some contain Auer bodies; variant M_3 contains few granules; peripheral bilobal blasts	≈ 100%	∅	∅	∅	MPO ⊕ and CD 13 ⊕ and CD 33⊕ and normally CD 34 ⊖ and HLA-DR ⊖
M_4	Acute myelomono-cytic leukemia; 30–80% of bone marrow blasts are myeloblasts, pro-myelocytes, and myelocytes; 20% are monocytes; vari-ant M_4 eosinophilia; additional imma-ture eosinophils with dark granules	≥ 3%	∅	+ > 20%	+	Mixed M 1/ M 2 and M 5

Table **14** Continued

FAB type*			Peroxidase	PAS	α-Naph-thyl-acetat-eesterase	Naph-thyl-ASD-esterase	Immuno-phenotype
M₅	a)	Acute mono-blastic leuke-mia; monoblasts predominant in the blood and bone marrow	±	∅	+++ > 80%	+++	CD 13/CD 33/ CD 65/CD 14/ CD64 ⊕/⊖ and HLA-DR ⊖⊕
	b)	Acute mono-cytic leukemia; monocytes in the process of maturation pre-dominante	±	∅	+++	+++	
M₆		Acute erythroid leukemia; 50% of bone marrow blasts are erythropoietic, 30% myeloblasts		∅	∅	∅	Erythroblasts Gly A ⊕ and CD 36 ⊕ Myeloblasts MPO/CD 13/CD 33/CD 65s ⊕/⊖ and CD 14 ⊖
M₇		Acute megakaryo-cytic leukemia; very polymorphic, some-times vacuolated blasts, some with cytoplastic blebs, sometimes aggre-gated with throm-bocytes	∅	±	±	±	CD 13/CD 33 ⊖/⊕ und CD 41 ⊕ oder CD 61 ⊕

* French American British Classification (FAB) 1976/85
** A biphenotypic leukemia must be considered a possibility if several additional lymphoblas-tic markers are present
PAS Periodic acid-Schiff reaction

Chromosome analysis provides important information. In practice, however, the diagnosis of acute leukemia is still based on morphological criteria.

However, where the possibilities of modern therapeutic and prognostic methods are fully accessible, new laboratory procedures based on genetic and molecular biological testing procedures form part of the diagnostic work-up of AML. The current WHO classification takes account of these new methods, placing genetic, morphological, and anamnestic findings in a hierarchical order (Table **15**).

 According to the new WHO classification, blasts account for more than 20% of cells in acute myeloid leukemia (in contradistinction to myelo-dysplasias).

Table **15** WHO classification of AML

AML with specific cytogenetic trans-locations	– With t(8;21) (q22; q22), AML 1/ETO – Acute promyelocytic leukemia (AML M3 with t(15;17) (q22; q11-12) and variants, PML/RAR-α – With abnormal bone marrow eosinophils and (inv16) (p13;q22) or to t(16;16) (p13; q22); CBFβ/MYH 11 – With 11q23 (MLL) anomalies
AML with dysplasia in *more than 1 cell line* (2 or 3 cell lines affected)*	– With preceding myelodysplastic/myeloproliferative syndrome – Without preceding myelodysplastic syndrome
Therapy-induced AML und MDS	– After treatment with alkylating agents – After treatment with epipodophyllotoxin – Other triggers
AML that does not fit any of the other categories	– AML, minimal differentiation – AML without cell maturation – AML with cell maturation – Acute myelomonocytic leukemia – Acute monocytic leukemia – Acute erythroid leukemia – Acute megakaryoblastic leukemia – Acute panmyelosis with myelofibrosis – Myelosarcoma/chloroma – Acute biphenotypic leukemia**

*   The dysplasia must be evident in at least 50% of the bone marrow cells and in 2–3 cell lines.
** Biphenotypic leukemias should be classified according to their immunophenotypes. They are grouped between acute lymphocytic and acute myeloid leukemias.

Acute Myeloid Leukemias (AML)

Morphological analysis makes it possible to group the predominant leukemic cells into myeloblasts and promyeloblasts, monocytes, or atypical (lympho)blasts. A morphological subclassification of these main groups was put forward in the French–American–British (FAB) classification (Table **14**).

> ! In practical, treatment-oriented terms, the most relevant factor is whether the acute leukemia is characterized as myeloid or lymphatic.

Including the very rare forms, there are at least 11 forms of myeloid leukemia.

Acute Myeloblastic Leukemia (Type M_0 through M_2 in the FAB Classification). Morphologically, the cell populations that dominate the CBC and bone marrow analyses (Fig. 31) more or less resemble myeloblasts in the course of normal granulopoiesis. Differences may be found to varying degrees in the form of coarser chromatin structure, more prominently defined nucleoli, and relatively narrow cytoplasm. Compared with lymphocytes (micromyeloblasts), the analyzed cells may be up to threefold larger. In a good smear, the transformed cells can be distinguished from lymphatic cells by their usually reticular chromatin structure and its irregular organization. Occasionally, the cytoplasm contains crystalloid azurophilic needle-shaped primary granules (Auer bodies). Auer bodies (rods) are conglomerates of azurophilic granules. A few cells may begin to display promyelocytic granulation. Cytochemistry shows that from stage M_1 onward, more than 3% of the blasts are peroxidase-positive.

Characteristics of Acute Leukemias

Age of onset: Any age.
Clinical findings: Fatigue, fever, and signs of hemorrhage in later stages.
Lymph node and mediastinal tumors are typical only in ALL.
Generalized involvement of all organs (sometimes including the meninges) is always present.
CBC and laboratory: Hb ↓, thrombocytes ↓, leukocytes usually strongly elevated (~ 80%) but sometimes decreased or normal.
In the differential blood analysis, blasts predominate (morphologies vary).
Beware: Extensive urate accumulation!
Further diagnostics: Bone marrow, cytochemistry, immunocytochemistry, cytogenetics, and molecular genetics.
Differential diagnosis: Transformed myeloproliferative syndrome (e.g., CML) or myelodysplastic syndrome.
Leukemic non-Hodgkin lymphomas (incl. CLL).
Aplastic anemias.
Tumors in the bone marrow (carcinomas, but also rhabdomyosarcoma).
Course, therapy: Usually rapid progression with infectious complications and bleeding.
Immediate efficient chemotherapy in a hematology facility; bone marrow transplant may be considered, with curative intent.

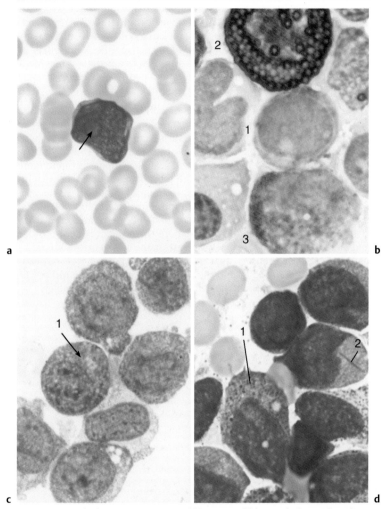

Fig. **31** Acute leukemia, M_0–M_2. **a** Undifferentiated blast with dense, fine chromatin, nucleolus (arrow), and narrow basophilic cytoplasm without granules. This cell type is typical of early myeloid leukemia (M_0–M_1); the final classification is made using cell surface marker analysis (see Table **14**). **b** The peroxidase reaction, characteristic of cells in the myeloid series, shows positive ($\geq 3\%$) only for stage M_1 leukemia and higher. The image shows a weakly positive blast (1), strongly positive eosinophil (2), and positive myelocyte (3). **c** and **d** Variants of M_2 leukemia. Some of the cells already contain granules (1) and crystal-like Auer bodies (2).

Acute Promyelocytic Leukemia (FAB Classification Type M_3 and M_{3v}). The characteristic feature of the cells, which are usually quite large with variably structured nuclei, is extensive promyelocytic granulation. Auer rods are commonly present. Cytochemistry reveals a positive peroxidase reaction for almost all cells. All other reactions are nonspecific. Acute leukemia with predominantly bilobed nuclei is classified as a variant of M_3 (M_{3v}). The cytoplasm may appear either ungranulated (M_3) or very strongly granulated (M_{3v}).

Acute Myelomonocytic Leukemia (FAB Classification Type M_4). Given the close relationship between cells in the granulopoietic and the monocytopoietic series (see p. 3), it would not be surprising if the these two systems showed a common alteration in leukemic transformation. Thus, acute myelomonocytic leukemia shows increased granulocytopoiesis (up to more than 20% myeloblasts) with altered cell morphologies, together with increased monocytopoiesis yielding more than 20% monoblasts or promonocytes. Immature myeloid cells (atypical myelocytes to myeloblasts) are found in peripheral blood in addition to monocyte-related cells. Cytochemically, the classification calls for more than 3% peroxidase-positive and more than 20% esterase-positive blasts in the bone marrow. M_4 is similar to M_2; the difference is that in the M_4 type the monocyte series is strongly affected. In addition to the above characteristics, the **M_4Eo** variant shows abnormal eosinophils with dark purple staining granules.

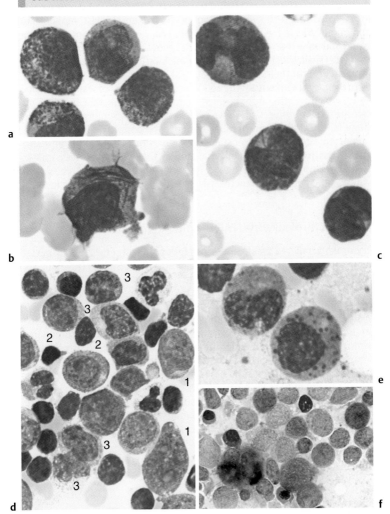

Fig. **32** Acute leukemia M3 and M4. **a** Blood analysis in promyelocytic leukemia (M3): copious cytoplasmic granules. **b** In type M3, multiple Auer bodies are often stacked like firewood (so-called faggot cells). **c** Blood analysis in variant M3v with dumbbell-shaped nuclei. Auer bodies **d** Bone marrow cytology in acute myelomonocytic leukemia M4: in addition to myeloblasts (1) and promyelocytes (2) there are also monocytoid cells (3). **e** In variant M4Eo abnormal precursors of eosinophils with dark granules are present. **f** Esterase as a marker enzyme for the monocyte series in M4 leukemia.

Acute Monocytic Leukemia (FAB Classification Types M$_{5a+b}$). Two morphologically distinct forms of acute monocytic leukemias exist, monoblastic and monocytic. In the *monoblastic* variant M$_{5a}$, blasts predominate in the blood and bone marrow. The blast nuclei show a delicate chromatin structure with several nucleoli. Often, only the faintly grayish-blue stained cytoplasm hints at their derivation.

In *monocytic* leukemia (type M$_{5b}$), the bone marrow contains promonocytes, which are similar to the blasts in monocytic leukemia, but their nuclei are polymorphic and show ridges and lobes. Some promonocytes show faintly stained azurophilic granules. The peripheral blood contains monocytoid cells in different stages of maturation which cannot be distinguished with certainty from normal monocytes. Both types are characterized by strong positive esterase reactions in over 80% of the blasts, whereas the peroxidase reactivity is usually negative, or positive in only a few cells.

Acute Erythroleukemia (FAB Classification Type M$_6$)

Erythroleukemia is a malignant disorder of both cell series. It is suspected when mature granulocytes are virtually absent, but blasts (myeloblasts) are present in addition to nucleated erythrocyte precursors, usually erythroblasts (for morphology, see p. 33). The bone marrow is completely overwhelmed by myeloblasts and erythroblasts (more than 50% of cells in the process of erythropoiesis). Bone marrow cytology and cytochemistry confirm the diagnosis. Sporadically, some cases show granulopenia, erythroblasts, and severely dedifferentiated blasts, which correspond to immature red cell precursors (proerythroblasts and macroblasts).

The *differential diagnosis* in cases of cytopenia with red blood cell precursors found in the CBC must include bone marrow carcinosis, in which the bone marrow–blood barrier is destroyed and immature red cells (and sometimes white cells) appear in the bloodstream. Bone marrow cytology and/or bone marrow histology clarifies the diagnosis. Hemolysis with hypersplenism can also show this constellation of signs.

Fig. **33**   Acute leukemia M$_5$ and M$_6$. **a** In monoblastic leukemia M$_{5a}$, blasts with a ▶ fine nuclear structure and wide cytoplasm dominate the CBC. **b** Seemingly mature monocytes in monocytic leukemia M$_{5b}$. **c** Homogeneous infiltration of the bone marrow by monoblasts (M$_{5a}$). Only residual granulopoiesis (arrow). **d** Same as **c** but after esterase staining. The stage M$_{5a}$ blasts show a clear positive reaction (red stain). There is a nonspecific-esterase (NSE)-negative promyelocyte.

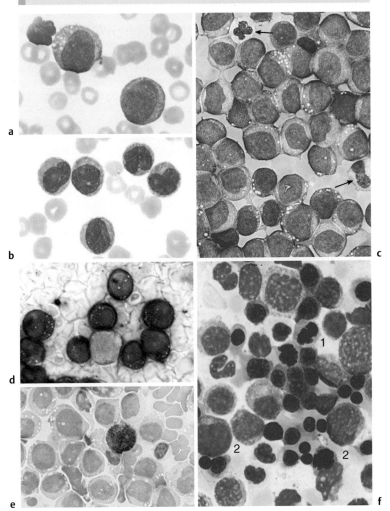

Fig. **33** **e** Same as **c** Only the myelocyte in the center stains peroxidase-positive (brown tint); the monoblasts are peroxidase-negative. **f** In acute erythrocytic leukemia (M_6) erythroblasts and myeloblasts are usually found in the blood. This image of bone marrow cytology in M_6 shows increased, dysplastic erythropoiesis (e.g., 1) in addition to myeloblasts (2).

Acute Megakaryoblastic Leukemia (FAB Classification Type M₇)

This form of leukemia is very rare in adults and occurs more often in children. It can also occur as "acute myelofibrosis," with rapid onset of tricytopenia and usually small-scale immigration into the blood of de-differentiated medium-sized blasts without granules. Bone marrow harvesting is difficult because the bone marrow is very fibrous. Only bone marrow histology and marker analysis (fluorescence-activated cell sorting, FACS) can confirm the suspected diagnosis.

The *differential diagnosis*, especially if the spleen is very enlarged, should include the megakaryoblastic transformation of CML or osteomyelosclerosis (see pp. 112 ff.), in which blast morphology is very similar.

AML with Dysplasia

The WHO classification (p. 94) gives a special place to AML with dysplasia in two to three cell series, either as primary syndrome or following a myelodysplastic syndrome (see pp. 106) or a myeloproliferative disease (see pp. 114 ff.).

Criteria for dysgranulopoiesis: ≥50% of all segmented neutrophils have no granules or very few granules, or show the Pelger anomaly, or are peroxidase-negative.

Criteria for dyserythropoiesis: ≥50% of the red cell precursor cells display one of the following anomalies: karyorrhexis, megaloblastoid traits, more than one nucleus, nuclear fragmentation.

Criteria for dysmegakaryopoiesis: ≥50% of at least six megakaryocytes show one of the following anomalies: micromegakaryocytes, more than one separate nucleus, large mononuclear cells.

Hypoplastic AML

Sometimes (mostly in the mild or "aleukemic" leukemias of the FAB or WHO classifications), the bone marrow is largely empty and shows only a few blasts, which usually occur in clusters. In such a case, a very detailed analysis is essential for a differential diagnosis versus aplastic anemia (see pp. 148 f.).

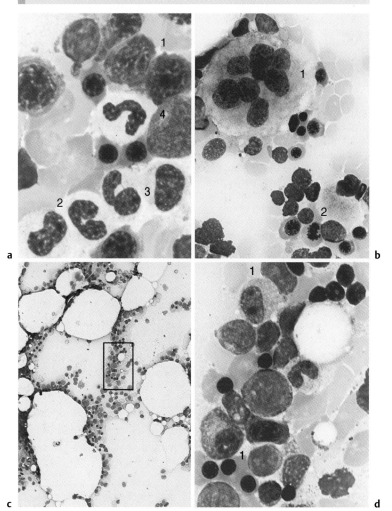

Fig. **34** AML with dysplasia and hypoplastic AML. **a** AML with dysplasia: megalo-blastoid (dysplastic) erythropoiesis (1) and dysplastic granulopoiesis with Pelger-Huët forms (2) and absence of granulation in a myelocyte (3). Myeloblast (4). **b** Multiple separated nuclei in a megakaryocyte (1) in AML with dysplasia. Dys-erythropoiesis with karyorrhexis (2). **c** and **d** Hypoplastic AML. **c** Cell numbers be-low normal for age in the bone marrow. **d** Magnification of the area indicated in **c**, showing predominance of undifferentiated blasts (e.g., 1).

Acute Lymphoblastic Leukemia (ALL)

ALL are the leukemias in which the cells do not morphologically resemble myeloblasts, promyelocytes, or monocytes, nor do they show the corresponding cytochemical pattern. Common attributes are a usually slightly smaller cell nucleus and denser chromatin structure, the grainy consistency of which can be made out only with optimal smear technique (i.e., very light). The classification as ALL is based on the (often remote) similarities of the cells to lymphocytes or lymphoblasts from lymph nodes, and on their immunological cell marker behavior. Insufficiently close morphological analysis can also result in possible confusion with chronic lymphocytic leukemia (CLL), but cell surface marker analysis (see below) will correct this mistake. Advanced diagnostics start with peroxidase and esterase tests on fresh smears, performed in a hematology laboratory, together with (as a minimum) immunological marker studies carried out on fresh heparinized blood samples in a specialist laboratory. The detailed differentiation provided by this cell surface marker analysis has prognostic implications and some therapeutic relevance especially for the distinction to bilineage leukemia and AML (Table **16**).

Table **16**   Immunological classification of acute bilineage leukemias (adapted from Bene MC et al. (1995) European Group for the Immunological Characterization of Leukemias (EGIL) 9: 1783–1786)

Score	B-lymphoid	T-lymphoid	Myeloid
2	CytCD79a*	CD3(m/cyt)	MP0
	Cyt IgM	anti-TCR	
1	CD19	CD2	CD117
	CD20	CD5	CD13
	CD10	CD8	CD33
		CD10	CD65
0.5	TdT	TdT	CD14
	CD24	CD7	CD15
		CD1a	CD64

* CD79a may also be expressed in some cases of precursor T-lymphoblastic leukemia/lymphoma.

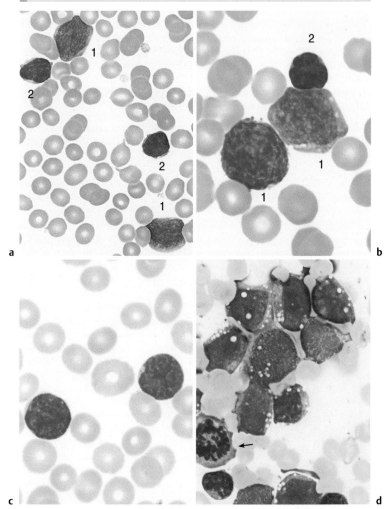

Fig. **35** Acute lymphocytic leukemias. **a** Screening view: blasts (1) and lymphocytes (2) in ALL. Further classification of the blasts requires immunological methods (common ALL). **b** Same case as **a** . The blasts show a dense, irregular nuclear structure and narrow cytoplasm (cf. mononucleosis, p. 69). Lymphocyte (2). **c** ALL blasts with indentations must be distinguished from small-cell non-Hodgkin lymphoma (e.g., mantle cell lymphoma, p. 77) by cell surface marker analysis. **d** Bone marrow: large, vacuolated blasts, typical of B-cell ALL. The image shows residual dysplastic erythropoietic cells (arrow).

105

Myelodysplasia (MDS)

Clinical practice has long been familiar with the scenario in which, after years of *bone marrow insufficiency* with a more or less pronounced deficit in all three cell series (*tricytopenia*), patients pass into a phase of insidiously increasing blast counts and from there into frank leukosis —although the evolution may come to a halt at any of these stages. The transitions between the forms of myelodysplastic syndromes are very fluid, and they have the following features in common:

➤ *Anemia, bicytopenia, or tricytopenia* without known cause.
➤ *Dyserythropoiesis* with sometimes pronounced erythrocyte anisocytosis; in the bone marrow often megaloblastoid cells and/or ring sideroblasts.
➤ *Dysgranulopoiesis* with pseudo-Pelger-Huët nuclear anomaly (hyposegmentation) and hypogranulation (often no peroxidase reactivity) of segmented and band granulocytes in blood and bone marrow.
➤ *Dysmegakaryopoiesis* with micromegakaryocytes.

The FAB classification is the best-known scheme so far for organizing the different forms of myelodysplasia (Table **17**).

Table **17**   Forms of myelodysplasia

Form of myelodysplasia	Blood analysis	Bone marrow
RA = refractory anemia	Anemia (normo-chromic or hyper-chromic); possibly pseudo-Pelger granulo-cytes; blasts ≤ 1 %	Dyserythropoiesis (marginal dysgranulo-poiesis and dysmega-karyopoiesis > 10 %) < 5 % blasts
RAS = refractory anemia with ring sidero-blasts (≑ aquired idiopathic sideroblastic anemia, p. 137)	Hypochromic and hyperchromic erythro-cytes side by side, sometimes discrete thrombopenia and leukopenia; pseudo-Pelger cells	More than 15 % of the red cell precursors are ring sideroblasts; blasts < 5 %
RAEB = refractory anemia with excess of blasts	Often thrombocyto-penia in addition to anemia; blasts < 5 %, monocytes < 1000/μl, pseudo-Pelger syndrome	Erythropoietic hyper-plasia (with or without ring sideroblasts); 5–20 % blasts

Cont. p. 108

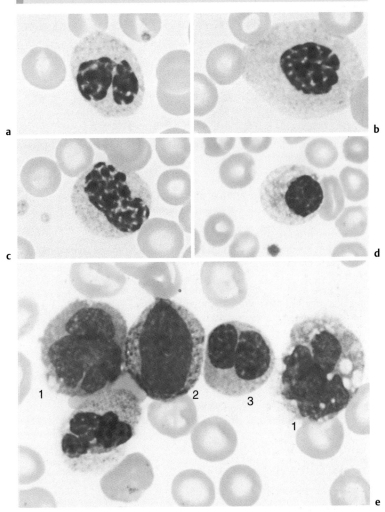

Fig. **36** Myelodysplasia and CMML. **a–d** Different degrees of abnormal maturation (pseudo-Pelger type); the nuclear density can reach that of erythroblasts (**d**). The cytoplasmic hypogranulation is also observed in normal segmented granulocytes. These abnormalities are seen in myelodysplasia or after chemotherapy, among other conditions. **e** Blood analysis in CMML: monocytes (1), promyelocyte (2), and pseudo-Pelger cell (3). Thrombocytopenia.

Table **17** Continued

Form of myelodysplasia	Blood analysis	Bone marrow
CMML = chronic myelo-monocytic leukemia	Blasts < 5 %, mono-cytes > 1000/µl, pseudo-Pelger syn-drome	Hypercellular, blasts < 20 %, elevated pro-monocytes
RAEB in transformation (RAEB_t) *	Similar to RAEB but > 5 % blasts	Blasts 20–30 % (some cells contain Auer bodies)

* In the WHO classification, the category RAEB_t would belong to the category of acute myeloid leukemia.

The new WHO classification of myelodysplastic syndromes defines the differences in cell morphology even more precisely than the FAB classification (Table **18**).

For the criteria of dysplasia, see page 106.

The "5q- syndrome" is highlighted as a specific type of myelodysplasia in the WHO classification; in the FAB classification it would be a subtype of RA and RAS. A macrocytic anemia, the 5q- syndrome manifests with normal or increased thrombocyte counts while the bone marrow contains megakaryocytes with hyposegmented round nuclei (Fig. **37 b**).

Naturally, *bone marrow analysis* is of particular importance in the myelodysplasias.

Table **18**   WHO classification of myelodysplastic syndromes

Disease*	Dysplasia**	Blasts in peripheral blood	Blasts in the bone marrow	Ring sidero-blasts in the bone marrow	Cytogenetics
5q- syndrome	Usually only E	< 5 %	< 5 %	< 15 %	5q only
RA	Usually only DysE	< 1 %	< 5 %	< 15 %	Variable
RARS	Usually only DysE	None	< 5 %	≥ 15 %	Variable
RCMD	2–3 lines	Rarely	< 5 %	< 15 %	Variable
RCMD-RS	2–3 lines	Rarely	< 5 %	≥ 15 %	Variable
RAEB-1	1–3 lines	< 5 %	5–9 %	< 15 %	Variable
RAEB-2	1–3 lines	5–19 %	10–19 %	< 15 %	Variable
CMML-1	1–3 lines	< 5 %	< 10 %	< 15 %	Variable
CMML-2	1–3 lines	5–19 %	10–19 %	< 15 %	Variable
MDS-U	1 cell lineage	None	< 5 %	< 15 %	Variable

* RA = refractory anemia; RARS = refractory anemia with ring sideroblasts; RCMD = refractory cytopenia with more than one dysplastic cell line; RCMD-RC = refractory cytopenia with more than one dysplastic lineage and ring sideroblasts; RAEB = refractory anemia with elevated blast count; CMML = chronic myelomonocytic leukemia, persistent monocytosis (more than 1×10^9/l) in peripheral blood; MDS-U = MDS, unclassifiable. ** Dysplasia in granulopoiesis = Dys G, in erythropoiesis = DysE, in megakaryopoiesis = DysM, multilineage dysplasia = two cell lines affected; trilineage dysplasia (TLD) = all three lineage show dysplasia.

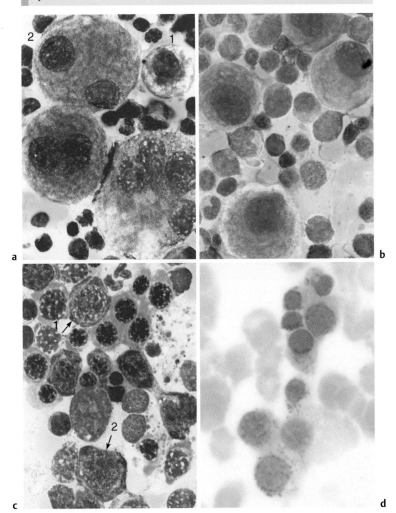

Fig. 37 Bone marrow analysis in myelodysplasia. **a** Dysmegakaryopoiesis in myelodysplastic syndrome (MDS). Relatively small disk-forming megakaryocytes (1) and multiple singular nuclei (2) are often seen. **b** Mononuclear megakaryocytes (frequent in 5 q-syndrome). **c** Dyserythropoiesis. Particularly striking is the coarse nuclear structure with very light gaps in the chromatin (arrow 1). Some are megaloblast-like but coarser (arrow 2). **d** Iron staining of the bone marrow (Prussian blue) in myelodysplasia of the RARS type: dense iron granules forming a partial ring around the nuclei (ring sideroblasts).

109

Prevalence of Polynuclear (Segmented) Cells (Table 19)

Neutrophilia without Left Shift

For clarity, conditions in which mononuclear cells (lymphocytes, monocytes) predominate were in the previous section kept distinct from hematological conditions in which cells with segmented nuclei and, in some cases, their precursors predominate. Leukocytosis with a predominance of segmented neutrophilic granulocytes without the less mature forms is called *granulocytosis* or *neutrophilia*.

Table **19**   Diagnostic work-up for anomalies in the white cell series with polynucleated (segmented) cells predominating

Clinical findings	Hb	MCH	Leuko-cytes	Segmented cells (%)	Lympho-cytes (%)	Other cells
Acute temperature, possibly focal signs	n	n	↑	↑	↓	Left shift
Patient smokes heavily (no splenomegaly)	n/↑	n	↑	↑	↓	∅
Slowly developing fatigue, spleen ↑	↓/n	↓/n	↑	↑	↓	Left shift
Slowly developing fatigue, spleen ↑	↓	↓	n/↑/↓	n/↑/↓	↓	Normoblasts, left shift
÷	↑ ↑	n	↑	↑	↓	Some normoblasts
Pruritus or exanthema	n	n	n/↑	n	n	↑ Eosinophils

Diagnostic steps proceed from left to right. | The next step is usually unnecessary; → the next step is obligatory.

Causes of Neutrophilia

➤ All kinds of stress
➤ Pregnancy
➤ Connective tissue diseases
➤ Tissue necrosis, e.g., after myocardial or pulmonary infarction
➤ Acidosis of various etiologies, e.g., nephrogenic diabetes insipidus
➤ Medications, drugs, or noxious chemicals, such as

– Nicotine	– Barbiturates
– Corticosteroids	– Lithium
– Adrenaline	– Streptomycin
– Digitalis	– Sulfonamide
– Allopurinol	

Throm-bocytes	Electro-phore-sis	Tentative diagnosis	Evidence/advanced diagnostics	Bone marrow	Ref. page
n	n	**Acute bacterial infection (possibly with leukemoid reaction)**	Search for disease focus		p. 112
n/ ↑	n	**Smoker's leukocytosis**	Anamnesis	In progressive disease: bone marrow analysis (DD myelo-proliferative disease)	p. 112
n/ ↑ / ↓	n	**Chronic myeloid leukemia (CML)**	Cytogenetics, *BCR-ABL*	Complete bone marrow analysis, all fractions	p. 116
n/ ↑ / ↓	n	**Osteomyelo-sclerosis**	Tear-drop-shaped erythrocytes	Often dry tap → bone mar-row histology	p. 122
n/ ↑	n	**Polycythemia with concom-itant leuko-cytosis**			p. 162
n	n	**Reactive eosinophilia**	Search for disease focus/allergen		p. 124

Reactive Left Shift

A relative left shift in the granulocyte series means *less mature forms in excess of 5% band neutrophils*; the preceding, less differentiated cell forms are included and all transitional forms are taken into account. This left shift almost always indicates an increase in new cell production in this cell series. In most cases, it is associated with a raised total leukocyte count. However, since total leukocyte counts are subject to various interfering factors that can also alter the cell distribution, *left shift without leukocytosis* can occur, and has no further diagnostic value. At best, if no other explanations offer, a left shift without leukemia can prompt investigation for splenomegaly, which would have prevented elevation of the leukocyte count by increased sequestration of leukocytes as in hypersplenism.

In evaluating the magnitude of a left shift, the basic principle is that the more immature the cell forms, the more rarely they appear; and that there is a continuum starting from segmented granulocytes and sometimes reaching as far as myeloblasts. Accordingly, a moderate left shift of medium magnitude may include myelocytes and a severe left shift may go as far as a few promyelocytes and (very rarely) myeloblasts, all depending on how fulminant the triggering process is and how responsive the individual. The term "pathological left shift" (for a left shift that includes promyelocytes and myeloblasts) is inappropriate, because such observations can reflect a very active *physiological* reaction, perhaps following a "leukemoid reaction" with pronounced left shift and leukocytosis.

Causes of Reactive Left Shift

Left shift occurs regularly in the following situations:

➤ Bacterial infections (including miliary tuberculosis),
➤ Nonbacterial inflammation (e.g., colitis, pancreatitis, phlebitis, and connective tissue diseases)
➤ Cell breakdown (e.g., burns, liver failure, hemolysis)

Left shift sometimes occurs in the following situations:

➤ Infection with fungi, mycoplasm, viruses, or parasites
➤ Myocardial or pulmonary infarction
➤ Metabolic changes (e.g., pregnancy, acidosis, hyperthyroidism)
➤ Phases of compensation and recuperation (hemorrhages, hemolysis, or after medical or radiological immunosuppression).

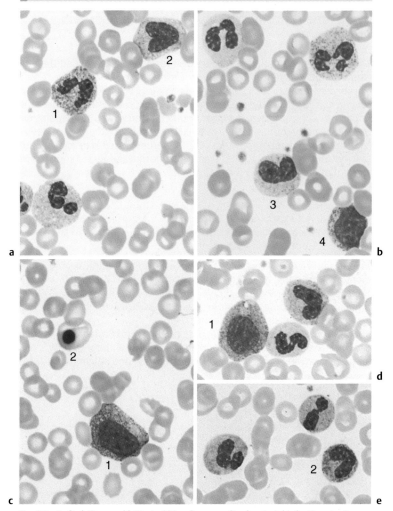

Fig. **38** Left shift. **a** and **b** Typical blood smear after bacterial infection: toxic granulation in a segmented granulocyte (1), monocyte with gray–blue cytoplasm (2), metamyelocyte (3), and myelocyte (4). **c** Blood analysis in sepsis: promyelocyte (1) and orthochromatic erythroblast (2). Thrombocytopenia. **d** and **e** Reactive left shift as far as promyelocytes (1). Particularly striking are the reddish granules in a band neutrophilic granulocyte (2).

Chronic Myeloid Leukemia and Myeloproliferative Syndrome (Chronic Myeloproliferative Disorders, CMPD)

The chronic myeloproliferative disorders (previously also called the myeloproliferative syndromes) include *chronic myeloid leukemia* (CML), *osteomyelosclerosis* (OMS), *polycythemia vera* (PV) and *essential thrombocythemia* (ET). Clearly, noxious agents of unknown etiology affect the progenitor cells at different stages of differentiation and trigger chronic malignant proliferation in the white cell series (CML), the red cell series (PV), and the thrombocyte series (ET). Sometimes, they lead to concomitant synthesis of fibers (OMS). Transitional forms and mixed forms exist particularly between PV, ET, and OMS.

> The chronic myeloproliferative disorders encompass chronic autonomous disorders of the bone marrow and the embryonic blood-generating organs (spleen and liver), which may involve one or several cell lines.

The common attributes of these diseases are onset in middle age, development of splenomegaly, and slow disease progression (Table **20**).

In 95 % of cases, *CML* shows a specific chromosome aberration (Philadelphia chromosome with a specific *BCR-ABL* translocation) and may make the transition into a blast crisis.

PV and *ET* often show similar traits (high thrombocyte count or high Hb) and have a tendency to secondary bone marrow fibrosis. *OMS* is primarily characterized by fibrosis in bone marrow and splenomegaly (see p. 122).

Table **20** Clinical characteristics and differential diagnostic criteria in chronic myeloproliferative disease

	CML (see p. 116)	PV (see p. 162)	OMS (see p. 122)	ET (see p. 170)
Spleno-megaly	+	No	+	No
Changes in the CBC for granulopoie-sis and/or erythropoie-sis	Leukocytosis with left shift, eosinophilia, *basophilia* !!	Leukocytosis, hematocrit ↑ !!	Tear-drop-shaped eryth-rocytes, left shift in the granulopoiesis, normoblasts	No
Thrombo-cytes	(↑)	(↑) Giant forms	↓ to (↑)	> 450 000/ µl ! giant forms
Bone marrow cytology	Very hyper-cellular, basophilia, megakaryo-cytes, and eosinophilia ↑	Markedly hypercellular, erythropoie-sis ↑	In most cases dry tap	Mega-karyo-cytes clearly elevated and arranged in nests
Bone marrow histology	Granulopoie-sis ↑ , mega-karyocytes ↑	Number of cells ↑	Advanced fibrosis !	Mega-karyo-cytes clearly elevated, arranged in nests
Philadelphia chromosome	Yes!	No	No	No
Other chro-mosomal alterations	In the accel-eration phase and blast cri-sis	del (20q), +8, +9, +1q, and others	-7, +8, +9, +1q, and others	Very rare
Alkaline Leukocyte-phosphatase (ALP)	↓ ↓ !	↑ ↑	Normal to ↑	Normal to ↑
Vitamin B$_{12}$ > 900 pg/ml	↑	↑	Normal	Normal

Characteristics of CML

Age of onset: Any age. Peak inicidence about 50 years.

Clinical findings: Slowly developing fatigue, anemia; in some cases palpable splenomegaly; no fever.

CBC: Leukocytosis and a left shift in the granulocyte series; possibly Hb ↓, thrombocytes ↓ or ↑.

Advanced diagnostics: Bone marrow, cytogenetics, and molecular genetics (Philadelphia chromosome and *BCR-ABL* rearrangement).

Differential diagnosis: Reactive leukocytoses (alkaline phosphatase, trigger?); other myeloproliferative disorders (bone marrow, cytogenetics, alkaline phosphatase).

Course, therapy: Chronic progression. Acute transformation after years. New, curative drugs are currently under development. Evaluate the possibility of a bone marrow transplant (up to age approx. 60 years).

Steps in the Diagnosis of Chronic Myeloid Leukemia

Left-shift leukocytosis in conjunction with usually low-grade anemia, thrombocytopenia or thrombocytosis (which often correlates with the migration of small megakaryocyte nuclei into the blood stream), and clinical splenomegaly is typical of CML. LDH and uric acid concentrations are elevated as a result of the increased cell turnover.

The average "typical" cell composition is as follows (in a series analyzed by Spiers): about 2% myeloblasts, 3% promyelocytes, 24% myelocytes, 8% metamyelocytes, 57% band and segmented neutrophilic granulocytes, 3% basophils, 2% eosinophils, 3% lymphocytes, and 1% monocytes.

In almost all cases of CML the hematopoietic cells display a marker chromosome, an anomalously configured chromosome 22 (*Philadelphia chromosome*). The translocation responsible for the Philadelphia chromosome corresponds to a special fusion gene (*BCR-ABL*) that can be determined by polymerase chain reaction (PCR) and fluorescence in situ hybridization (FISH).

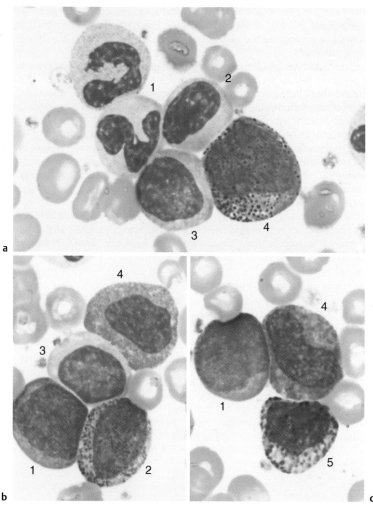

Fig. **39** CML. **a** Blood analysis in chronic myeloid leukemia (chronic phase): segmented neutrophilic granulocytes (1), band granulocyte (2) (looks like a metamyelocyte after turning and folding of the nucleus), myelocyte with defective granulation (3), and promyelocyte (4). **b** and **c** Also chronic phase: myeloblast (1), promyelocyte (2), myelocyte with defective granulation (3), immature eosinophil (4), and basophil (5) (the granules are larger and darker, the nuclear chromatin denser than in a promyelocyte).

117

Bone Marrow Analysis in CML. In many clinical situations, the findings from the CBC, the *BCR-ABL* transformation and the enlarged spleen unequivocally point to a diagnosis of CML. Analysis of the bone marrow should be performed because it provides a series of insights into the disease processes.

Normally, the cell density is considerably elevated and granulopoietic cells predominate in the CBC. Cells in this series mature properly, apart from a slight left shift in the chronic phase of CML. CML differs from reactive leukocytoses because there are *no signs of stress*, such as toxic granulation or dissociation in the nuclear maturation process.

Mature neutrophils may occasionally show pseudo-Pelger forms (p. 43) and the *eosinophilic* and, especially, *basophilic granulocyte* counts are often elevated. The proportion of cells from the red blood cell series decreases. Histiocytes may store glucocerebrosides, as in Gaucher syndrome (pseudo-Gaucher cells), or lipids in the form of sea-blue precipitates (sea-blue histiocytes after Romanowsky staining).

Megakaryocytes are usually increased and are often present as *micromegakaryocytes*, with one or two nuclei which are only slightly larger than those of promyelocytes. Their cytoplasm typically shows clouds of granules, as in the maturation of thrombocytes.

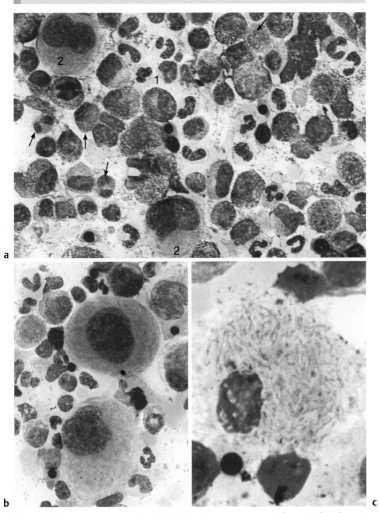

a

b

c

Fig. **40** Bone marrow cytology in CML. **a** Bone marrow cytology in the chronic phase: increased cell density due to increased, left-shifted granulopoiesis, e.g., promyelocyte nest (1) and megakaryopoiesis (2). Eosinophils are increased (arrows), erythropoiesis reduced. **b** Often micromegakaryocytes are found in the bone marrow cytology. **c** Pseudo-Gaucher cells in the bone marrow in CML.

Blast Crisis in Chronic Myeloid Leukemia

During the course of CML with or without therapy, regular monitoring of the differential smear is particularly important, since over periods of varying duration the relative proportions of blasts and promyelocytes increases noticeably. When the blast and promyelocyte fractions together make up 30%, and at the same time Hb has decreased to less than 10 g/dl and the thrombocyte count is less than 100 000/µl, an incipient acute blast crisis must be assumed. this blast crisis is often accompanied or preceded by a *markedly increased basophil count*. Further blast expansion—usually largely recalcitrant to treatment—leads to a clinical picture not always clearly distinguishable from acute leukemia. If in the chronic phase the disease was "latent" and medical treatment was not sought, enlargement of the spleen, slight eosinophilia and basophilia, and the occasional presence of normoblasts, together with the overwhelming myeloblast fraction, are all signs indicating CML as the cause of the blast crisis.

As in AML, in two-thirds of cases cytological and immunological tests are able to identify the blasts as myeloid. In the remaining one-third of cases, the cells carry the same markers as cells in ALL. This is a sign of dedifferentiation. A final megakaryoblastic or a final erythremic crisis is extremely rare.

Bone marrow cytology is particularly indicated when clinical symptoms such as fatigue, fever, and painful bones suggest an acceleration of CML which is not yet manifest in the CBC. In such a case, bone marrow analysis will frequently show a much more marked shift to blasts and promyelocytes than the CBC. A proportion of more than 20% immature cell fractions is sufficient to diagnose a blast crisis.

The prominence of other cell series (erythropoiesis, thrombopoiesis) is reduced. The basophil count may be elevated.

A bone marrow aspiration may turn out to be empty (sicca) or scarcely yield any material. This suggests fibrosis of the bone marrow, which is frequently a complicating symptom of long-standing disease. Staining of the fibers will demonstrate this condition in the bone marrow histology.

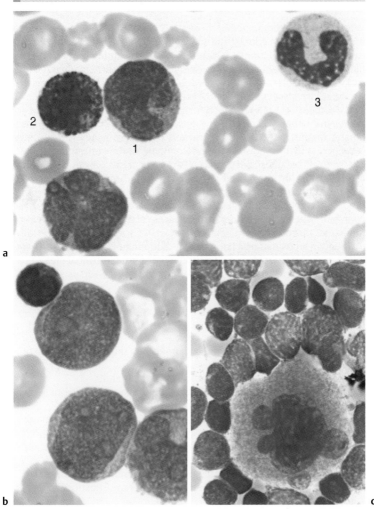

Fig. **41** Acute blast crisis in CML. **a** Myeloblasts (1) with somewhat atypical nuclear lobes. Basophilic granulocyte (2) and band granulocyte (3). Thrombocytopenia. The proliferation of basophilic granulocytes often precedes the blast crisis. **b** Myeloblasts in an acute CML blast crisis. Typical sand-like chromatin structure with nucleoli. A lymphocyte. **c** Bone marrow cytology in acute CML blast crisis: blasts of variable sizes around a hyperlobulated megakaryocyte (in this case during a lymphatic blast crisis).

121

Osteomyelosclerosis

When anemia accompanied by moderately elevated (although sometimes reduced) leukocyte counts, thrombocytopenia or thrombocytosis, clinically evident splenic tumor, left shift up to and including sporadic myeloblasts, and eosinophilia, the presence of a *large proportion of red cell precursors* (normoblasts) in the differential blood analysis, osteomyelosclerosis should be suspected. *BCR-ABL* gene analysis is negative.

Pathologically, osteomyelosclerosis usually originates from megakaryocytic neoplasia in the bone marrow and the embryonic hematopoietic organs, particularly spleen and liver, accompanied by fibrosis (= sclerosis) that will eventually predominate in the surrounding tissue. The central role of cells of the megakaryocyte series is seen in the giant thrombocytes, or even small coarsely structured megakaryocyte nuclei without cytoplasm, that migrate into the blood stream and appear in the CBC. OMS can be a primary or secondary disease. It may arise during the course of other myeloproliferative diseases (often polycythemia vera or idiopathic thrombocythemia).

Tough, fibrous material hampers the sampling of bone marrow material, which rarely yields individual cells. This in itself contributes to the bone marrow analysis, allowing differential diagnosis versus reactive fibroses (parainfectious, paraneoplastic).

Characteristics of OMS

Age of onset: Usually older than 50 years.
Clinical findings: Signs of anemia, sometimes skin irritation, drastically enlarged spleen.
CBC: Usually tricytopenia, normoblasts, and left shift.
Further diagnostic procedures: Fibrous bone marrow (bone marrow histology), when appropriate and *BCR-ABL* (always negative).
Differential diagnosis: Splenomegaly in cases of lymphadenoma or other myeloproliferative diseases: bone marrow analysis.
Myelofibrosis in patients with metastatic tumors or inflammation: absence of splenomegaly.
Course, therapy: Chronic disease progression; transformation is rare. If there is splenic pressure: possibly chemotherapy, substitution therapy.

Further myeloproliferative diseases are described together with the relevant cell systems: polycythemia vera (see p. 162) and essential thrombocythemia (see p. 170).

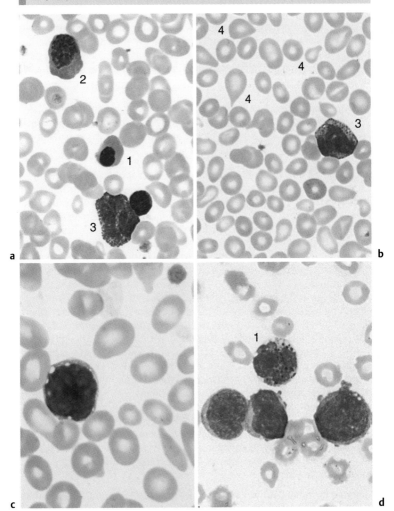

Fig. **42** Osteomyelosclerosis (OMS). **a** and **b** Screening of blood cells in OMS: red cell precursors (orthochromatic erythroblast = 1 and basophilic erythroblast = 2), basophilic granulocyte (3), and teardrop cells (4). **c** Sometimes small, dense megakaryocyte nuclei are also found in the blood stream in myeloproliferative diseases. **d** Blast crisis in OMS: myeloblasts and segmented basophilic granulocytes (1).

123

Elevated Eosinophil and Basophil Counts

In accordance with their physiological role, an *increase in eosinophils* ($> 400/\mu l$, i.e. for a leukocyte count of 6000, more than 8% in the differential blood analysis) is usually due to *parasitic attack* (p. 5). In the Western hemisphere, parasitic infestations are investigated on the basis of stool samples and serology.

> **!** *Strongyloides stercoralis* in particular causes strong, sometimes extreme, elevation of eosinophils (may be up to 50%). However, eosinophilia of variable degree is also seen in ameba infection, in lambliasis (giardiasis), schistosomiasis, filariasis, and even malaria.

Bacterial and viral infections are both unlikely ever to lead to eosinophilia except in a few patients with scarlet fever, mononucleosis, or infectious lymphocytosis. The second most common group of causes of eosinophilia are *allergic conditions:* these include asthma, hay fever, and various dermatoses (urticaria, psoriasis). This second group also includes drug-induced hypersensitivity with its almost infinitely multifarious triggers, among which various antibiotics, gold preparations, hydantoin derivatives, phenothiazines, and dextrans appear to be the most prevalent. Eosinophilia is also seen in *autoimmune diseases*, especially in scleroderma and panarteritis. All *neoplasias* can lead to "paraneoplastic" eosinophilia, and in Hodgkin's disease it appears to play a special role in the pathology, although it is nevertheless not always present.

A specific *hypereosinophilia syndrome* with extreme values (usually $> 40\%$) is seen clinically in association with various combinations of splenomegaly, heart defects, and pulmonary infiltration (Loeffler syndrome), and is classified somewhere between autoimmune diseases and myeloproliferative syndromes. Of the leukemias, CML usually manifests moderate eosinophilia in addition to its other typical criteria (see p. 114). When moderate eosinophilia dominates the hematological picture, the term *chronic eosinophilic leukemia* is used. Acute, absolute predominance of eosinophil blasts with concomitant decrease in neutrophils, erythrocytes, and thrombocytes suggests the possibility of the very rare *acute eosinophilic leukemia.*

Elevated Basophil Counts. Elevation of segmented basophils to more than 2–3% or $150/\mu l$ is rare and, in accordance with their physiological role in the immune system regulation, is seen inconsistently in *allergic reactions* to food, drugs, or parasites (especially filariae and schistosomes), i.e., usually in conditions in which eosinophilia is also seen. *Infectious diseases* that may show basophilia are tuberculosis and chickenpox; *metabolic diseases* where basophilia may occur are myxedema and hyperlipidemia. Autonomic proliferations of basophils are part of the myeloproliferative

Eosinophilia and basophilia are usually accompanying phenomena in reactive and myeloproliferative disorders, especially
CML

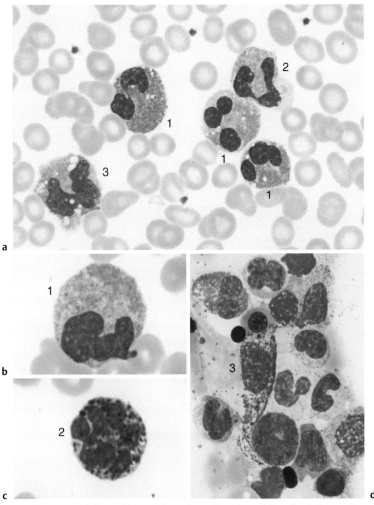

Fig. **43** Eosinophilia and basophilia. **a** Screening view of blood cells in reactive
eosinophilia: eosinophilic granulocytes (1), segmented neutrophilic granulocyte
(2), and monocyte (3) (reaction to bronchial carcinoma). **b** and **c** The image shows
an eosinophilic granulocyte (1) and a basophilic granulocyte (2) (clinical osteomyelosclerosis). **d** Bone marrow in systemic mastocytosis: tissue mast cell (3),
which, in contrast to a basophilic granulocyte, has an unlobed nucleus, and the cytoplasm is wide with a tail-like extension. Tissue mast cells contain intensely basophilic granules.

125

pathologies and can develop to the extent of being termed "chronic basophilic leukemia." In the very rare *acute basophilic leukemia*, the cells in the basophilic granulocyte lineage mature in the bone marrow only to the stage of promyelocytes, giving a picture similar to type M_3 AML (p. 98).

Being an expression of idiopathic disturbance of bone marrow function, elevated basophil counts are a relatively constant phenomenon in *myeloproliferative syndromes* (in addition to the specific signs of these diseases), especially in CML. Acute basophilic leukemia is extremely rare; in this condition, some of the dedifferentiated blasts contain more or less basophilic granules.

The tissue-bound analogs of the segmented basophils, the tissue mast cells, can show benign or malignant cell proliferation, including the (extremely rare) acute mast cell leukemia (Table **21**).

Table **21** Different forms of benign and malignant proliferation of tissue mast cells

Clinical picture	Clinical diagnosis	Evidence
In childhood, solitary or multiple skin nodules, some brownish	Localized mastocytosis	Histology
↓ Sometimes transition		
Diffuse brownish papules, with urticaria on irritation	Urticaria pigmentosa	Typical clinical picture
↓		
Hyperpigmented spots, papules and/or dermographism; histamine symptoms: flushing, headache, pruritus, abdominal spasms, shock	Systemic mastocytosis	Histology
↓		
Malignant transformation, possibly with osteolysis, enlarged lymph nodes, splenomegaly, hepatomegaly	Malignant mastocytosis*	Histology
↓		
Migration of leukemic cells to peripheral blood	Acute mast cell leukemia	CBC (bone marrow)

* May occur *de novo* without preceding stages and without skin involvement.

Erythrocyte and Thrombocyte Abnormalities

Clinically Relevant Classification Principle for Anemias: Mean Erythrocyte Hemoglobin Content (MCH)

In current diagnostic practice, erythrocyte count and hemoglobin content (grams per 100 ml) in whole blood are determined synchronously. This allows calculation of the hemoglobin content per individual erythrocyte (mean corpuscular hemoglobin, MCH) using the following simple formula (p. 10):

$$\frac{Hb\ (g/dl) \cdot 10}{Ery\ (10^6/\mu l)}$$

The mean cell volume, hematocrit, MCH, and erythrocyte size can be used for various calculations (Table **22**; methods p. 10, normal values Table **2**, p. 12). Despite this multiplicity of possible measures, however, in routine diagnostic practice the differential diagnosis in cases of low Hb concentration or low erythrocyte counts relies above all on the MCH, and most forms of anemia can safely be classified by reference to the normal data range of 26–32 pg Hb/cell (1.61–1.99 fmol/cell) as *normochromic* (within the normal range), *hypochromic* (below the), or *hyperchromic* (above the norm). The *reticulocyte count* (p. 11) provides important additional pathophysiological information. Anemias with increased erythrocyte production (*hyper-regenerative anemias*) suggest a high reticulocyte count, while anemias with diminished erythrocyte production (*hyporegenerative anemias*) have low reticulocyte counts (Table **22**).

It should be noted that hyporegenerative anemias due to iron or vitamin deficiency can rapidly display hyper-regeneration activity after only a short course of treatment with iron or vitamin supplements (up to the desirable "reticulocyte crisis").

The practical classification of anemia starts with the MCH:

— 26–32 pg = normochromic
— Less than 26 pg = hypochromic
— More than 32 pg = hyperchromic

Hypochromic Anemias

Iron Deficiency Anemia

Most anemias are hypochromic. Their usual cause is iron deficiency from various causes (Fig. **44**). To distinguish quickly between real iron deficiency and an iron distribution disorder, *iron* and *ferritin* levels should be determined.

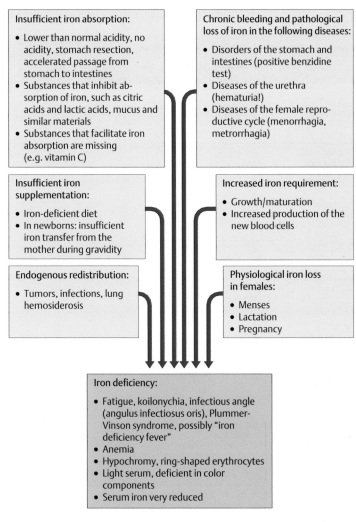

Insufficient iron absorption:

- Lower than normal acidity, no acidity, stomach resection, accelerated passage from stomach to intestines
- Substances that inhibit absorption of iron, such as citric acids and lactic acids, mucus and similar materials
- Substances that facilitate iron absorption are missing (e.g. vitamin C)

Chronic bleeding and pathological loss of iron in the following diseases:

- Disorders of the stomach and intestines (positive benzidine test)
- Diseases of the urethra (hematuria!)
- Diseases of the female reproductive cycle (menorrhagia, metrorrhagia)

Insufficient iron supplementation:

- Iron-deficient diet
- In newborns: insufficient iron transfer from the mother during gravidity

Increased iron requirement:

- Growth/maturation
- Increased production of the new blood cells

Endogenous redistribution:

- Tumors, infections, lung hemosiderosis

Physiological iron loss in females:

- Menses
- Lactation
- Pregnancy

Iron deficiency:

- Fatigue, koilonychia, infectious angle (angulus infectiosus oris), Plummer-Vinson syndrome, possibly "iron deficiency fever"
- Anemia
- Hypochromy, ring-shaped erythrocytes
- Light serum, deficient in color components
- Serum iron very reduced

Fig. **44** The most important reasons for iron deficiency (according to Begemann)

Table **22**   Diagnostic findings and work-up for the most important disorders of the red cell series

Clinical findings	Hb	MCH	Erythrocyte morphology	Reticulocytes	Leukocytes	Segmented nuclei (%)	Lymphocytes (%)	Other cells	Thrombocytes
Fatigue, pallor (dysphagia)	↓	↓	Ring-shaped erythrocytes, anisocytosis	↓	n	n	n	-	n/↑
Possibly fever, weight loss	↓	↓	Anisocytosis, poikilocytosis	↓	n/↑	n	n	Possibly eosinophils ↑ monocytes ↑ left shift	n
Diffuse symptoms	↓	↓/n/↑	All sizes, dimorphic	↓	n/↓	n	n	-	n/↓
Acute hemorrhage	↓	n	n	n	n	(↑)	(↓)	-	n/↓ /↑
Subjaundice	↓	n	n or pathol., possibly spherocytes	↑ ↑	n/↓	n	n	Possibly normoblasts	n/↓
Spleen ↑	↓	↓	Target cells	↑	n	n	n	Possibly normoblasts	n
Paller possibly infections and bleeding tendency	↓	n	n	↓↓	↓	↓	↑	Possibly monocytes ↑	↓↓
Pallor possibly alcohol history	↓	↑	Macrocytes, megalocytes	↓	↓	↓	↑	Possibly hypersegmented granulocytes, possibly normoblasts	↓/n
Plethora, possibly spleen	↑	n	n	n	n/↑	n	n	-	n/↑
Acute bleeding tendency	↓	n	n	(↑)	n	n	n	-	↓↓

Diagnostic steps proceed from left to right. I The next step is usually unnecessary; ⋮ the next step is optional; → the next step is obligatory. n = normal value, ↓ = lower than normal, ↑ = elevated, ( ) = test not relevant, BSG = erythrocyte sedimentation rate.

BSG	Electro-phoresis	Iron	Ferritin and others	Trans-ferrin	Tentative diagnosis	Evidence/ further diag-nostics	Bone marrow	Ref. page
n	n	↓	Ferritin ↓	↑	**Iron deficiency anemia**	Determine source of bleed-ing; check iron absorption	Erythropoiesis ↑ sideroblasts ↓, iron in macro-phages ↓	p. 132
↑	? α₂↑ γ↑	↓	Ferritin n/↑	↓	**Acquired/sec-ondary anemia (infectious/ toxic, paraneo-plastic)**	Search for trigger	Erythropoiesis ↓, sideroblasts ↓ iron in macro-phages ↑	p. 134
n	n	↑	n/↑	↓	**Sideroachrestic anemia, myelodysplasia**	⟶	Erythropoiesis ↑, ring sideroblasts present	p. 106
n	n	n/↓	–	n/↑	**Anemia due to hemorrhaging**	Search for source and reason for hemorrhages	(Erythropoiesis ↑)	p. 140
n	n	n	Hapto-globu-lin ↓↓	(n/↓)	**Hemolytic anemia**	Osmotic resistance, Coombs test,	(Erythropoiesis ↑ , right shift) increased storage of iron	p. 140
n	n	n	Hapto-globu-lin ↓↓		**Especially: thalassemia**	Hb electro-phoresis and further tests		p. 138
↑	n	↑/(n)	n/↑	(↓/n)	**Aplastic ane-mia or bone marrow carci-nosia**	Search for trig-ger or tumor	Hypoplasia of all cell series, or car-cinoma cells	p. 146, 148, 150
n	n	n/↑	Vitamin B₁₂ folic acid ↓	(↓)	**Megaloblastic anemia**	Gastroscopy, determination of antibodies, possibly Schilling test	Erythropoietic megaloblasts	p. 152
n/↓	n	↓	↑	↑	**Polyeythemia, DD: hypergam-maglobuline-mia**	ALP, progress-ion	Erythropoiesis ↑	p. 162
n	n	↓	duration of hemor-rhaging ↑↑ PTT n	–	**Thrombocyto-penic purpura (ITP)**	Search for trig-gers, possibly also for anti-bodies	Elevated mega-karyocyte count	p. 166

Table **23**   Normal ranges for physiological iron and its transport proteins

	Old units	SI units
Serum iron		
Newborns	150–200 µg/dl	27–36 µmol/l
Adults		
Female	60–140 µg/dl	11–25 µmol/l
Male	80–150 µg/dl	14–27 µmol/l
TIBC	300–350 µg/dl	54–63 µmol/l
Transferrin	250–450 µg/dl	2.5–4.5 g/l
Serum ferritin	30–300 µg/l (15–160 µg/l premenopausal)	

TIBC = Total iron binding capacity.

This usually renders determination of transferrin and total iron binding capacity (TIBC) unnecessary. If samples are being sent away to a laboratory, it is preferable to send serum produced by low-speed centrifugation, since the erythrocytes in whole blood can become mechanically damaged during shipment and may then release iron. Table **23** shows the variation of serum iron values according to gender and age.

It is important to note that *acute* blood loss causes normochromic anemia. Only *chronic bleeding* or earlier serious acute blood loss leads to iron deficiency manifested as hypochromic anemia.

Iron Deficiency and Blood Cell Analysis Focusing on the erythrocyte morphology is the quickest and most efficient way to investigate hypochromic anemia when the serum iron has dropped below normal values. In hypochromic anemia with iron and hemoglobin deficiency (whether due to insufficient iron intake or an increased physiological iron requirement), *erythrocyte size and shape* does not usually vary much (see Fig. **45**). Only in advanced anemias (from approx. 11 g/dl, equivalent to 6.27 mmol/l Hb) are relatively small erythrocytes (microcytes) with reduced MCV and MCH and grayish stained basophilic erythrocytes (polychromatic erythrocytes) seen, indicating inadequate hemoglobin content. Cells with the appearance of relatively large polychromatic erythrocytes are reticulocytes. The details of their morphology can be seen after supravital staining (p. 141). A few target cells (p. 139) will be seen in conditions of severe iron deficiency.

In severe hemoglobin deficiency (< 8 g/dl, equivalent to 4.96 mmol/l) the residual hemoglobin is found mostly at the peripheral edge of the erythrocyte, giving the appearance of a *ring-shaped erythrocyte*.

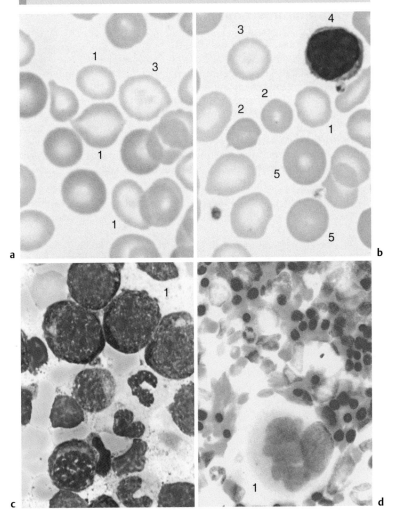

Fig. **45** Iron deficiency anemia. **a** and **b** Erythrocyte morphology in iron deficiency anemia: ring-shaped erythrocytes (1), microcytes (2) faintly visible target cells (3), and a lymphocyte (4) for size comparison. Normal-sized erythrocytes (5) after transfusion. **c** Bone marrow cytology in iron deficiency anemia shows only increased hematopoiesis and left shift to basophilic erythroblasts (1). **d** Absence of iron deposits after iron staining (Prussian blue reaction). Megakaryocyte (1).

133

Hypochromic Infectious or Toxic Anemia (Secondary Anemia)

Among the various causes of lack of iron for erythropoiesis (see Fig. **44**, p. 129), a special situation is represented by the internal iron shift caused by "iron pull" of the reticuloendothelial system (RES) during *infections*, *toxic processes*, *autoimmune diseases*, and *tumors*. Since this anemia results from another disorder, it is also called *secondary* anemia. The MCH is hypochromic, or in rare instances, normochromic, and therefore erythrocyte morphology is particularly important to diagnosis. In contrast to exogenous iron deficiency anemias, the following phenomena are often observed, depending on the severity of the underlying condition:

➤ *Anisocytosis*, i.e., strong variations in the size of the erythrocytes, beyond the normal distribution. The result is that in almost every field view, some erythrocytes are either half the size or twice the size of their neighbors.

➤ *Poikilocytosis*, i.e., variations in the shape of the erythrocytes. In addition to the normal round shape, numbers of oval, or pear, or tear shaped cells are seen.

➤ *Polychromophilia*, the third phenomenon in this series of nonspecific indicators of disturbed erythrocyte maturation, refers to light gray-blue staining of the erythrocytes, indicating severely diminished hemoglobin content of these immature cells.

➤ *Basophilic cytoplasmic stippling* in erythrocytes is a sign of irregular regeneration and often occurs nonspecifically in secondary anemia.

The reticulocyte count is usually reduced in infectious or toxic anemia, unless there is concomitant hemolysis or acute blood loss.

Bone marrow analysis in secondary anemia usually shows reduced erythropoiesis and granulopoiesis with a spectrum of immature cells ("infectious/toxic bone marrow"). The information is so nonspecific that usually bone marrow aspiration is not performed. So long as all other laboratory methods are employed, bone marrow cytology is very rarely needed in cases of hypochromic anemia.

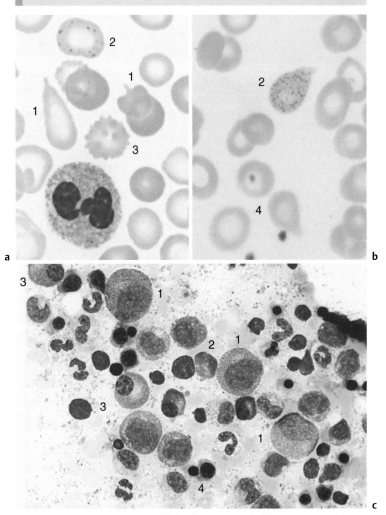

a

b

c

Fig. **46** Secondary anemia. **a** and **b** Erythrocyte morphology in secondary hypochromic anemia: the erythrocytes vary greatly in size (anisocytosis) and shape (1) (poikilocytosis), and show basophilic stippling (2). Burr cell (3), which has no specific diagnostic significance. Occasionally, the erythrocytes stain a soft gray–blue (4) (polychromasia). **c** Bone marrow cell overview in secondary anemia. Cell counts in the white cell series are elevated (promyelocytes = 1), eosinophils (2), and plasma cells (3); erythropoiesis is reduced (4).

Bone Marrow Cytology in the Diagnosis of Hypochromic Anemias

> ! So long as all other laboratory methods are employed, bone marrow cytology is very rarely needed in cases of hypochromic anemia.

Bone marrow cytology is rarely strictly indicated after all other available diagnostic methods have been exhausted (Table **22**, p. 130). However, in doubtful cases it can usually at least help to rule out malignant disease.

In *iron deficiency anemias* of the most various etiologies, erythropoiesis is stimulated in a compensatory fashion, and the distribution of the markers shows the expected increase in red cell precursors. The erythropoiesis to granulopoiesis ratio increases in favor of erythropoiesis from 1 : 3 to 1 : 2, but rarely further. The red cell series shows a left shift, i.e., there are more immature red cell precursors (erythroblasts and proerythroblasts) (for normal values, see Table **4**). Usually, these red cell precursors do not show any clearly atypical morphology, but the cytoplasm is basophilic even in normoblasts, according with the poor hemoglobinization. Iron staining of the bone marrow shows no sideroblasts (normoblasts containing iron granules), or only very few (< 10%, norm 30–40%). A constant finding in anemia stemming from exogenous iron deficiency is absence of iron in the macrophages of the bone marrow reticulum.

Megakaryocyte counts are almost always increased in iron deficiency due to chronic hemorrhaging, but can also show increased proliferation in iron deficiency from other causes (which can lead to increased thrombocyte counts in states of iron deficiency).

In *infectious or toxic (secondary) anemia*, unlike exogenous iron deficiency anemia, erythropoiesis tends to be somewhat suppressed. There is no left shift and no specific anomalies are present. Granulopoiesis predominates and often shows nonspecific "stress phenomena" and a dissociation of nuclear and cytoplasmic maturation (e.g., cytoplasm that is still basophilic with promyelocytic granules in mature, banded myelocyte nuclei).

Depending on the trigger of the anemia, the monocyte, lymphocyte, or plasma cell counts are often moderately increased, and megakaryocyte counts are occasionally slightly elevated. The important indicator is iron staining of the bone marrow. The "iron pull" of the RES leads to intensive iron storage in macrophages, while the red cell precursors are almost iron-free. However, combinations do exist, when a pre-existing iron deficiency means that the iron depositories are empty even in an infectious or toxic process. Moreover, not every secondary anemia is hypochromic. Where there is concomitant alcoholism or vitamin deficiency, secondary anemia may be normochromic or hyperchromic.

Hypochromic Sideroachrestic Anemias
(Sometimes Normochromic or Hyperchromic)

In a sideroachrestic anemia existing iron cannot be utilized (achrestic = useless). This is a suspected diagnosis when serum iron levels are raised or in the high normal range, and when the erythrocytes show *strong anisocytosis*, *poikilocytosis* (with reduced average MCV), *polychromophilia*, and in some cases also *basophilic stippling* (Fig. **46**). This suspicion can be further illuminated by *bone marrow analysis*. Unlike in infectious/toxic anemias, the red cell series is well represented. Iron staining of the bone marrow is the decisive diagnostic test, causing the iron-containing red precursor cells (sideroblasts) to stand out (hence the term "sideroblastic anemia.") The iron precipitates often collect in a ring around the nucleus ("ringed sideroblasts").

By far the majority of the "idiopathic sideroachrestic anemias," as they used to be called, are myelodysplasias (see p. 106). Only a few of them appear to be hereditary or have exogenous triggers (alcoholism, lead poisoning).

Hypochromic Anemia with Hemolysis

Thalassemias

A special form of hypochromic anemia mostly affecting patients of Mediterranean descent presents with normal erythrocyte count, decreased MCH, and clinical splenomegaly. The smear displays erythrocytes with central hemoglobin islands (*target cells*). These cells do not necessarily predominate in the CBC: the most revealing field views show at most 50% target cells in addition to clear anisocytosis and frequent basophilic stippling. Occasional *normoblasts* give a general indication of increased erythropoiesis. Although target cells are also nonspecific, since they can occur in such conditions as severe iron deficiency or obstructive jaundice, this overall picture should prompt hemoglobin electrophoresis. The sample consists of ACD-stabilized blood at 1 : 10 dilution. A significant increase in the HbA$_2$ fraction confirms a diagnosis of *thalassemia minor*, the heterozygous form of the disease. *Thalassemia major,* the homozygous variant, is far rarer and more serious. In this form of the disease, in addition to the target cells, the CBC shows a marked increase in red precursor cells. Hb-electrophoresis shows a predominance of HbF (the other hemolytic anemias are usually normochromic, see p. 140).

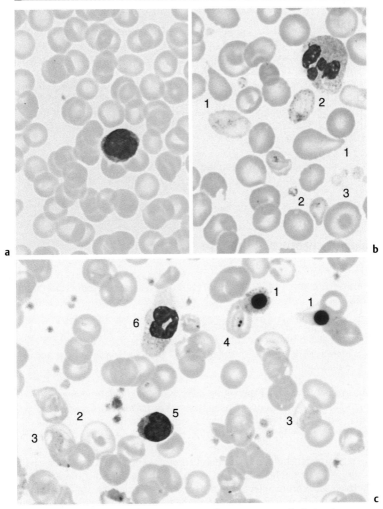

Fig. **47** Thalassemia. **a** Thalassemia minor: often no target cells, but an increase in the number of small erythrocytes (shown here in comparison with a lymphocyte), so that sometimes there is no anemia. **b** More advanced thalassemia minor: strong anisocytosis and poikilocytosis (1), basophilic stippling (2), and sporadic target cells (3). **c** Thalassemia major: erythroblasts (1), target cell (2), polychromatic erythrocytes (3), and Howell–Jolly bodies (4) (in a case of functional asplenia). Lymphocyte (5) and granulocyte (6).

Normochromic Anemias

Anemias where red cell hemoglobinization is normal (26–32 pg/dl, equivalent to 1.61–1.99 fmol/l) and average MCVs are normal (77–100 fl) can broadly be explained by three mechanisms: a) acute *blood loss* with sufficient metabolic reserves remaining; b) elevated *cell turnover* in which iron is reused as soon as it becomes free, so that hypochromia does not arise (this is typical of almost all *hemolytic anemias* except thalassemias; see p. 138); and c) *suppression* of cell production under conditions of normal iron supply (this is the group of *hypoplastic–aplastic anemias*, which have a variety of causes).

> **!** — In cases of acute blood loss: clinical findings, occult blood?
> — In hemolytic cases: reticulocytes ↑, haptoglobin ↓, possibly bilirubin ↑.
> — In bone marrow suppression: e.g. aplastic anemia, reticulocytes ↓.

Normochromic Hemolytic Anemias

Hemolytic anemias result from a shortened erythrocyte life span with insufficient compensation from increased erythrocyte production (Table **24**).

> **!** Usually, hematopoiesis in the bone marrow is increased in compensation, and, depending on the course of the disease, may make up for the accelerated cell degradation for all or some of the time by recycling the iron as it becomes free.

Accordingly, counts of the young, newly emerged erythrocytes (*reticulocytes)* are *always raised*, and usually sporadic *normoblasts* are found. Anemia proper often becomes apparent only in a "crisis" with acute, accelerated cell degradation, and reticulocyte counts increased up to more than 500%.

A common cellular phenomenon after extended duration of hemolytic anemia is the manifestation of macrocytic hypochromic disorders (p. 150), because the chronic elevation of hematopoietic activity can exhaust the endogenous folic acid reserves (*pernicious anemia*).

Bone marrow analysis shows both relative and absolute increases in erythropoietic activity: among the red cell precursors, in acute severe hemolysis the more immature forms often predominate more than in normal bone marrow, and in chronic hemolysis the maturer forms do (orthochromatic normoblasts). In addition, the normoblasts in hemolytic bone marrow often are markedly clustered (Fig. **48**), whereas in normal bone marrow they are more evenly dispersed (Fig. **18**).

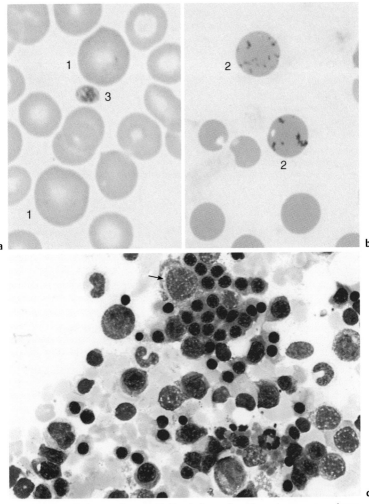

Fig. **48** Hemolytic anemia. **a** and **b** Newly formed erythrocytes appear as large, polychromatic erythrocytes (1) after Pappenheim staining (**a**); supravital staining (**b**) reveals spot-like precipitates (reticulocyte = 2). Thrombocyte (3). **c** Bone marrow cells in hemolytic anemia at low magnification: increased hematopoiesis with cell clusters. Orthochromatic erythroblasts predominate. A basophilic erythroblast shows loosened nuclear structure (arrow), a sign of secondary folic acid deficiency.

141

Table **24** Causes of the most common hemolytic anemias

	Special morphological features of erythrocytes	Further advanced diagnostics
Causes within the erythrocytes (corpuscular hemolyses)		
➤ Hereditary		
● Membrane abnormalities		
– Spherocytosis (see p. 144)	– Small spherocytes	Osmotic resistance
– Elliptocytosis	– Elliptocytes	
● Hemoglobin abnormalities		
– Thalassemia (see p. 138)	– Target cells	Hemoglobin electro-phoresis
– Sickle cell anemia (see p. 144)	– Sickle cells	
– Other rare hemoglobin-related disorders		
● Enzyme defects		
– Glucose-6-phosphate dehydrogenase	– Possibly Heinz bodies	Enzyme tests
– Pyruvate kinase and many others	– Macrocytes	
➤ Acquired		
● Paroxysmal nocturnal hemoglobinuria		Sucrose hemolysis test, absence of CD 55 (DAF) and CD 59
● Zieve syndrome	– Foam cells in the bone marrow	MIRL (membrane inhibitor of reactive lysis)
Causes outside the erythrocytes (extracorpuscular hemolyses)		
➤ Biosynthesis of antibodies		
● Isoantibodies (fetal erythro-blastosis, transfusion events)		Rh serology
● Warm autoantibodies		Coombs test
● Cold autoantibodies	– Autoagglutination	Coombs test, Cold agglutination titer
● Chemical-allergic antibodies (e.g., cephalosporin, methyl-dopa)		
➤ Physical or chemical noxae (e.g., after burns, heart valve replacement; heavy metal exposure, animal- or plant-derived poisons)	– Partially Heinz bodies	
➤ Microangiopathic hemolysis in hemolytic-uremic syndrome, thrombotic-thrombocytopenic purpura, bone marrow carci-noses	– Schizocytes, fragmen-tocytes (see p. 143)	Thrombocytes ↓ Liver, kidney
➤ Infection-related noxae (e.g. influenza, salmonella infection, malaria)	– For malaria pathogen (see p. 158)	Demonstration of pathogen
➤ Hypersplenism, e.g. lymphatic system disease, infections with splenomegaly, portal hyperten-sion		Cause of splenomegaly

Distribution pattern and shape of erythrocytes can be relevant in the diagnosis of hemolysis

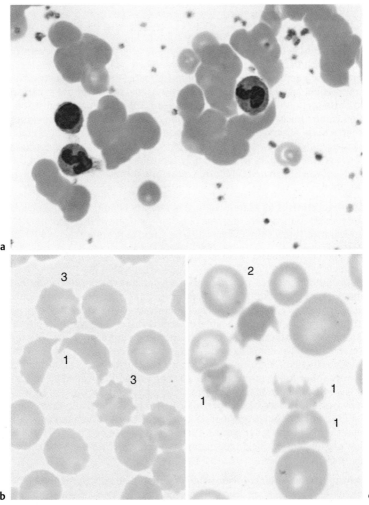

Fig. **49** Autoagglutination and fragmentocytes. **a** Clumps of erythrocytes. If this is the picture in all regions of the smear, an artifact is unlikely and serogenic (auto)agglutination should be suspected (in this case due to cryoagglutinins in mycoplasmic pneumonia). Thrombocytes are found between the agglutinated erythrocytes. **b** and **c** Conspicuous half-moon and egg-shell-shaped erythrocytes: fragmentocytosis in microangiopathic hemolytic anemia. Fragmentocytes (1), target cell (2), and echinocytes (3) (this last has no diagnostic relevance).

Cytomorphological Anemias with Erythrocyte Anomalies

Microspherocytosis This corpuscular form of hemolysis is characterized by dominant genetic transmission, splenomegaly, and a long uneventful course with occasional hemolytic crises. Blood analysis shows erythrocytes which appear strikingly small in comparison with leukocytes. The central light area is absent or only faintly visible, since they are spherical in cross-section rather than barbell-shaped. The abnormal size distribution can be measured in two dimensions and plotted using Price–Jones charts. Close observation of the morphology in the smear (Fig. **50**) is particularly important, because automated blood analyzers will determine a normal cell volume. The extremely reduced osmotic resistance of the erythrocytes (in the NaCl dilution series) is diagnostic. Coombs test is negative.

Stomatocytosis is an extremely rare hereditary condition. Stomatocytes are red cells with a median streak of pallor, giving the cells a "fish mouth" appearance. A few stomatocytes may be found in hepatic disease.

Hemoglobinopathies (see also thalassemia, p. 138). Target cells are frequently present (Fig. **47**).

In addition to target cells, smears from patients with *sickle cell anemia* may show a few sickle-shaped erythrocytes, but more usually these only appear under conditions of oxygen deprivation (Fig. **50**). (This can be achieved by covering a fresh blood droplet with a cover glass; a droplet of 2% $Na_2S_2O_4$ may be added). Sickle cell anemia is a dominant autosomal recessive hemoglobinopathy and is diagnosed by demonstrating the HbS band in Hb-electrophoresis. Homozygous patients with sickle cell anemia always suffer from chronic normocytic hemolysis. If provoked by oxygen deficiency or infections, severe crises may occur with clogging of the microvasculature by aggregates of malformed erythrocytes. Patients who are heterozygous for sickle cell anemia have the sickle cell trait but do not display the disease or its symptoms. These can, however, be triggered by very low oxygen tension. Sickle cell anemia is quite often combined with other hemoglobinopathies, such as thalassemia.

Schistocytosis (Fragmentocytosis) If, in acquired hemolytic anemia, some of the erythrocytes are fragmented and have various irregular shapes (eggshell, helmet, triangle, or crescent; Fig. **49**), this may be an indication of changes in the capillary system (microangiopathy), or else of disseminated intravascular coagulopathy (DIC). *Microangiopathic hemolytic anemias* develop in the course of thrombotic thrombocytopenic purpura (TTP, Moschcowitz disease) and its related syndromes: in children (hemolytic uremic syndrome, HUS); in pregnant women (HELLP syndrome); or in patients with bone marrow metastases from solid tumors.

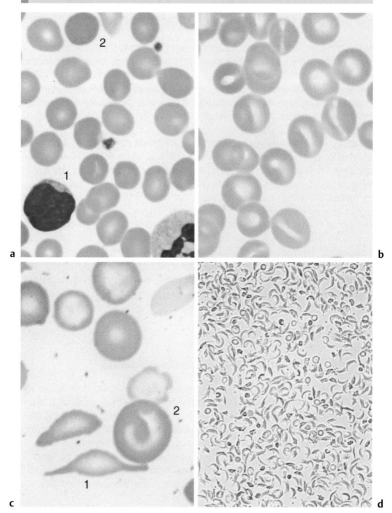

Fig. **50** Microspherocytes and sickle cells. All erythrocytes are strikingly small in comparison with lymphocytes (1) and lack a lighter center: these are microsphe-rocytes (diameter < 6 μm). Polychromatic erythrocyte (2). **b** Erythrocytes with an elongated rather than round lighter center: these are stomatocytes, which are rarely the cause of anemia. **c** Native sickle cells (1) are found only in homozygous sickle cell anemia, otherwise only target cells (2) are present. **d** Sickle cell test under reduced oxygen tension: almost all erythrocytes appear as sickle cells in the homozygous case presented here.

145

Normochromic Renal Anemia
(Sometimes Hypochromic or Hyperchromic)

Normochromic anemia should also suggest the possibility of renal insufficiency, which will always lead to anemia within a few weeks. In cases of chronic renal insufficiency it is always present and may reach Hb values as low as 6 g/dl. The anemia is caused by changes in the synthesis of erythropoietin, the hormone regulating erythropoiesis; measurement of serum erythropoietin is an important diagnostic tool. Erythrocyte life span is also slightly reduced.

Apart from poikilocytosis, the blood cells are morphologically unremarkable. The reticulocyte counts often remain normal. The bone marrow does not show any significant characteristic changes, and therefore serves no diagnostic purpose in this situation.

Anemias due to renal insufficiency are usually normochromic, but hypochromic or hyperchromic forms do occur. Hypochromic anemia is an indicator of the reactive process that has led to the renal insufficiency (e.g., pyelonephritis and glomerulonephritis), resulting in secondary hypochromic anemia. In addition, dialysis patients often develop iron deficiency. Chronic renal insufficiency can lead to folic acid deficiency, and dialysis therapy will reinforce this, explaining why hyperchromic anemias also occur in kidney disease.

Bone Marrow Aplasia

Pure Red Cell Aplasia (PRCA, Erythroblastopenia)

Erythroblastopenia in the sense of a purely aplastic condition in the red cell series is extremely rare. Diamond–Blackfan anemia (congenital hypoplastic anemia) is the congenital form of this disease. Acquired acute, transient infections in adults and children are usually caused by virus infections (parvovirus B19). Chronic acquired erythroblastophthisis is frequently associated with thymoma and has an autoimmune etiology.

Anemia in pure erythroblastophthisis is normochromic without significant changes in the CBC for white cells and thrombocytes. Naturally, the reticulocyte count is extremely low, close to zero.

In all these anemias, the bone marrow shows well-developed granulopoiesis and megakaryopoiesis, but erythropoiesis is (more or less) entirely lacking.

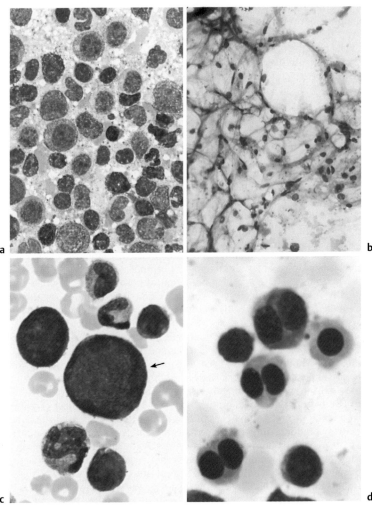

Fig. 51 Forms of bone marrow aplasia. **a** Bone marrow cytology in erythroblastopenia: only activated cells of the granulopoietic series are present. The megakaryopoiesis (not shown here) show no abnormalities. **b** Bone marrow aplasia: hematopoiesis is completely absent: only adipocytes and stroma cells are seen. **c** Giant erythroblast (arrow) in the bone marrow in acute parvovirus B19 infection. **d** Conspicuous binuclear erythroblasts in the bone marrow of a patient with congenital dyserythropoietic anemia (type II CDA).

147

The *differential diagnosis* in this context relates to very rare congenital dyserythropoietic anemias (CDA). These anemias manifest mostly in childhood or youth and may be normocytic or macrocytic. The bone marrow shows increased erythropoiesis with multinucleated erythroblasts, nuclear fragmentation, and cytoplasmic bridges. There are three types (type II carries the so-called HEMPAS antigen: *h*ereditary *m*ultinuclearity with *p*ositive *a*cidified *s*erum lysis test).

Aplasias of All Bone Marrow Series (Panmyelopathy, Panmyelophthisis, Aplastic Anemia)

A reduction in erythrocyte, granulocyte, and thrombocyte cell counts in these series, which may progress to zero, is far more common than pure erythroblastopenia and is always acquired (except in the rare pediatric Fanconi syndrome with obvious deformities).

Pathologically, this life-threatening disease is a result of damage to the hematopoietic stem cells, often by chemical toxins or, occasionally, viral infection. An autoimmune response of the T-lymphocytes also seems to play a role.

The term "panmyelopathy" is synonymous with "aplastic anemia" in the broader sense and with "panmyelophthisis."

The CBCs show the rapid progression of normochromic anemia and greatly reduced reticulocyte counts. Granulocyte counts gradually dwindle to zero, followed by the monocytes. Thrombocytes are usually also quite severely affected.

The remaining blood cells in all series appear normal, although naturally, given the presence of the noxious agents or intercurrent infections, they often show reactive changes (e.g., toxic granulations). The bone marrow aspirate for cytological analysis is often notable for poor yield of material, although a completely empty aspirate (dry tap) is rare.

The material obtained yields unfamiliar images in a smear (Fig. **51**). Frequently, strings and patches of reticular (stroma) cells from the bone marrow predominate, which normally are barely noticed in an aspirate. There are usually no signs of phagocytosis. Aside from the reticular cells, there are isolated lymphocytes, plasma cells, tissue basophils, and macrophages. Depending on the stage in the aplastic process, there may be residual hematopoietic cells. In some instances, the whole disease process is focal. For this reason, bone marrow histology must be performed whenever the cytological findings are insufficient or dubious in cases of tricytopenia of unknown cause.

Differential Diagnosis versus Reduction in Cell Counts in Several Series (Bicytopenia or Tricytopenia):

➤ After thorough analysis, most cytopenias with *hyperplasia* of the bone marrow have to be defined as *myelodysplasias* (p. 106), unless they are caused by accelerated cell degeneration (e.g., in hypersplenism).

➤ Cytopenia with bone marrow fibrosis points to myeloproliferative-type diseases (p. 114) or results from direct toxic or inflammatory agents.

➤ Cytopenia can of course also occur after *bone marrow infiltration* by malignant cells (carcinoma, sarcoma), which will not be contained in every bone marrow aspirate. This is why, when the diagnosis is uncertain, histological analysis should always be carried out.

➤ Cytopenia can also result from B_{12} or folic acid deficiency (but note the possibility of hyperchromic anemia, p. 152).

➤ Another cause of cytopenia is *expansion of malignant hematopoietic cells* in the bone marrow. This is easily overlooked if the malignant cells do not appear in the bloodstream, as in *plasmacytoma, lymphadenoma,* and *aleukemic leukemia* (leukemia without peripheral blasts).

➤ Cytopenia also develops of course after high-dose radiation or chemotherapy. In such cases it is not so much the CBC or bone marrow analysis as the exposure history that will allow the condition to be distinguished from the panmyelopathies described above.

➤ Cytopenia caused by *panmyelopathy mechanisms* (see preceding text; triggers shown in Table **25**).

Table **25** Substances, suspected or proven to cause panmyelopathy

Analgesics, antirheumatic drugs	Phenylbutazone, oxyphenbutazone, other nonsteroidal antirheumatic drugs, gold preparations, penicillamine
Antibiotics	Chloramphenicol, sulfonamide
Anticonvulsive drugs	Hydantoin
Thyrostatic drugs	Carbimazole/methimazole
Sedatives	Phenothiazines
Other medications	Cimetidine, tolbutamide
Insecticides	Hexachlorcyclohexane and other chlorinated hydrocarbons
Solvents	Benzene
Viruses	z. B. Hepatitis, CMV

In unexplained anemia, thrombocytopenia, or leukocytopenia, any possible triggers (Table **25**) must be discontinued or avoided. Panmyelophthisis or aplastic anemia is an acute disease that can only be overcome with aggressive treatment (glucocorticoids, cyclosporin, antilymphocyte globulin).

Bone Marrow Carcinosis and Other Space-Occupying Processes

Anemia resulting from bone marrow infiltration by growing, space-occupying tumor metastases can in principle be normochromic. However, under the indirect influence of the underlying disease, it tends more often to be hypochromic (secondary anemia).

Normoblasts in the differential blood analysis (Fig. **9 a**, p. 33) particularly suggest the possibility of bone marrow carcinosis, because their presence implies destruction of the bone marrow–blood barrier. Usually, bone marrow carcinosis leads eventually to lower counts in other cell series, especially thrombocytes.

 Bone metastases from malignant tumors rarely affect the bone *marrow* and hematopoiesis, and if they do, it is usually late. The most common metastases in bone *marrow* derive from small-cell bronchial carcinoma and breast cancer.

In the differential diagnosis, the effects of direct bone marrow infiltration must be distinguished from phenomena caused by microangiopathic hemolytic anemia (MHA) in the presence of tumor (p. 144). Carcinosis and MHA may of course coexist.

Bone marrow cytology in these situations tends to reveal a generally decreased density of hematopoietic cells and signs of reactive marrow as seen in secondary anemia (p. 134). Only in a few field views—often at the edge of the smear—will one occasionally encounter atypical cell elements which cannot be assigned with certainty to any of the hematopoietic blast families. The critical feature is their close arrangement in *clusters*. These atypical cells are at least as large as myeloblasts or proerythroblasts (e.g., in small-cell bronchial carcinoma), usually considerably larger. Tumor type cannot be diagnosed with certainty (except, e.g., melanoma). Bone marrow histology and possibly immunohistology tests must be performed if there is any doubt, or in the case of negative cytological findings or dry tap, since the clustered, focal character of metastases naturally means that they may not be obtained in every aspirate.

Thrombocytopenia with leukocytosis and erythroblasts in the peripheral blood: consider bone marrow carcinosis

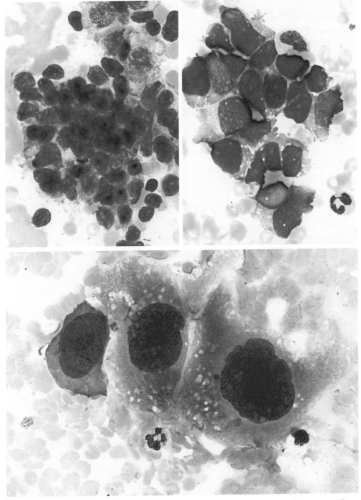

Fig. **52**   Bone marrow carcinosis. **a** and **b** Bone marrow smear at low magnification showing islands of infiltration by a homogeneous cell type (**a**), or, alternatively, by apparently different cell types which do, however, all display identical chromatin structure and cytoplasm: bone marrow carcinosis in breast carcinoma (**a**) or bronchial non-small-cell carcinoma (**b**). **c** Island of dedifferentiated cells in the bone marrow which cannot be assigned to any of the hematopoietic lineages: bone marrow carcinosis (here in a case of embryonal testicular cancer).

Hyperchromic Anemias

In patients with clear signs of anemia, e.g., a "sickly pallor," atrophic lingual mucosa, and sometimes also neurological signs of bathyanesthesia (loss of deep sensibility), even just a cursory examination of the blood smear may indicate the diagnosis. Marked poikilocytosis and anisocytosis are seen, and the large size of the erythrocytes is particularly conspicuous in comparison with the lymphocytes, whose diameter they exceed (megalocytes). These are the hallmarks of *macrocytic,* and, with respect to bone marrow cells, usually also *megaloblastic anemia,* with a mean cell diameter greater than 8 µm and a cell volume (MCV) usually greater than 100 µm^3. Mean cell Hb content (MCH) is more than 36 pg (1.99 fmol) and thus indicates *hyperchromic anemia.*

Only when there is severe pre-existing concomitant iron deficiency is a combination of macrocytic cells and hypochromic MCH possible ("dimorphic anemia").

Table **26**   Most common causes of hyperchromic anemias

Vitamin-B$_{12}$ deficiency	Folic acid deficiency
Nutritional deficits, e. g.	**Nutritional deficits**
– Goat milk	– Chronic abuse of alcohol
– Vegetarian diet	
– Alcoholism	
Impaired absorption	**Impaired absorption**
– Genuine pernicious anemia	– E. g., sprue (psilosis)
– Status after gastrectomy	**Increased requirement**
– Ileum resection	– Pregnancy
– Crohn disease	– Hemolytic anemia
– Celiac disease, sprue (psilosis)	**Interference/antagonism**
– Intestinal diverticulosis	– Phenylhydantoin
– Insufficiency of the exocrine pancreas	– Cytostatic antimetabolic drugs
– Fish tapeworm	– Trimethoprim (antibacterial combination drug)
	– Oral contrazeptives
	– Antidepressants
	– Alcohol

Although other rare causes exist (Table **26**), almost all patients with hyperchromic anemia suffer from *vitamin B$_{12}$* and/or *folic acid deficiency.* Since a deficiency of these essential metabolic building blocks suppresses DNA synthesis not only in erythropoiesis, but in the other cell series as well, over time more or less severe pancytopenia will develop.

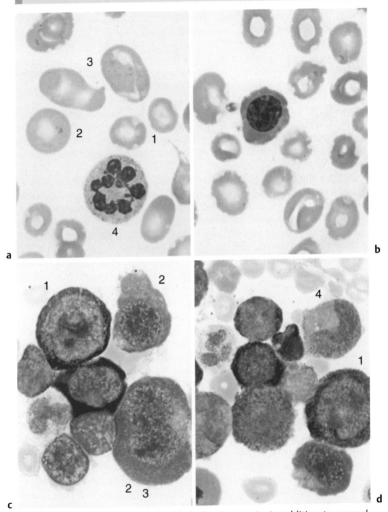

Conspicuous large erythrocytes suggest hyperchromic macro-cytic anemia, usually megaloblastic in the bone marrow

Fig. **53** Hyperchromic anemia. **a** Marked anisocytosis. In addition to normal-sized erythrocytes (1), macrocytes (2) and large ovoid megalocytes are seen (3). Hypersegmented granulocyte (4). **b** In hyperchromic anemia, red cell precursors may be released into the peripheral blood: here, a polychromatic erythroblast. **c** and **d** Bone marrow in megaloblastic anemia: slight (1) or marked (2) loosening up of the nuclear structure, in some cases with binuclearity (3). Giant forms of band granulocytes and metamyelocytes (4) are often present.

153

With hypersegmentation, i.e. >4–5 segments/nucleus, the segmented granulocytes show all the indications of a maturation disorder. In addition, the reticulocyte count is increased (but it may also be normal), and the iron content is elevated or normal.

> **!** Megaloblastic anemias show the same hematological picture whether they are caused by folic acid deficiency or by vitamin B_{12} deficiency.

Table **26** lists possible causes. It should be emphasized that "genuine" *pernicious anemia* is less common than megaloblastic anemia due to vitamin B_{12} deficiency. In pernicious anemia a stomach biopsy shows atrophic gastritis and usually also serum antibodies to parietal cells and intrinsic factor.

Among the causes of folic acid deficiency is chronic alcoholism (with insufficient dietary folic acid, impaired absorption, and elevated erythrocyte turnover). On the other hand, many alcoholics with normal vitamin B_{12} and folic acid levels develop severe hyperchromic anemia with a special bone marrow morphology, obviously with a pathomechanism of its own (pyridoxine [B_6] deficiency, among others).

In *megaloblastic anemia* (Fig. **53**) the cell density in the bone marrow is always remarkably high. Large to medium-sized blasts with round nuclei dominate the erythrocyte series. They are present in varying sizes, their chromatin is loosely arranged with a coarse "sandy" reticular structure, there are well-defined nucleoli, and the cytoplasm is very basophilic with a perinuclear lighter zone. These cells can be interpreted as proerythroblasts and macroblasts whose maturation has been disturbed. As these disturbed megaloblastic cells appear along a continuous spectrum from the less mature to the more mature, they are all referred to collectively as *megaloblasts*.

In the granylocytic series, anomalies become obvious at the myelocyte stage; characteristic giant cells with loosely structured nuclei develop which may tend to be classified as myelocytes/stab cells, but which in fact probably are myelocytes in which the maturation process has been disturbed. As in peripheral blood smears, segmented granulocytes are often hypersegmented. Megakaryocytes also show hypersegmentation of their nuclei or many individual nuclei. Iron staining reveals increased number of iron-containing reticular cells and sideroblasts, and a few ring sideroblasts may develop. All these changes disappear after vitamin B_{12} supplementation, after just three days in the erythrocyte series and within one week in the granulocyte series. In the differential diagnosis, in relation to the causes listed in Table **26**, the following should be highlighted: *toxic alcohol damage* (vacuolized proerythroblasts), *hemolytic anemia* (elevated reticulocyte count), *myelodysplasia* (for bone marrow morphology see Fig. **37**, p. 109).

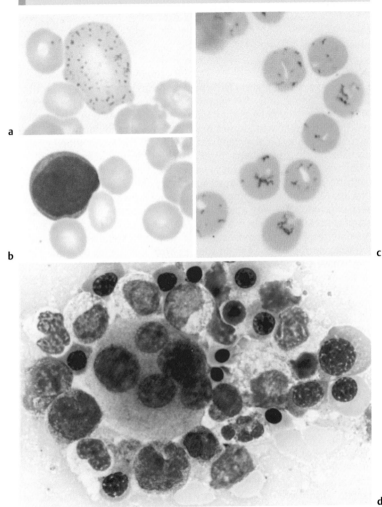

Fig. 54 Myelodysplastic syndrome (MDS) as differential diagnosis in hyperchromic anemia. **a** Strongly basophilic stippling in the cytoplasm of a macrocyte (in myelodysplasia). **b** Myeloblast with hyperchromic erythrocyte as an example of a myelodysplastic blood sample in the differential diagnosis versus hyperchromic anemia. **c** A high proportion of reticulocytes speaks against megaloblastic anemia and for hemolysis (in this case with an absence of pyruvate kinase activity). **d** Bone marrow in myelodysplasia (type RAEB), with clinical hyperchromic anemia.

Erythrocyte Inclusions

Erythrocytes normally show fairly homogeneous hemoglobinization after panoptic staining; only after supravital staining (p. 155) will the remains of their ribosomes show as *substantia granulofilamentosa* in the reticulocytes. Under certain conditions during the preparation of erythrocytes, aggregates of ribosomal material may be seen as basophilic stippling, also visible after Giemsa staining (Fig. **55 a**). This is normal in fetal and infant blood; in adults a small degree of basophilic stippling has nonspecific diagnostic value, like anisocytosis indicating only a nonspecific reactive process. Not until a large proportion of basophilic stippled erythrocytes is seen concomitantly with anemia does this phenomenon have diagnostic significance: thalassemia, lead poisoning, and sideroblastic anemia are all possibilities. Errant chromosomes from the mitotic spindle are sometimes found in normoblasts as small spheres with a diameter of about 1 μm, which have remained in the erythrocyte after expulsion of the nucleus and lie about as unevenly distributed Howell–Jolly bodies in the cytoplasm (Fig. **55 b**, **c**). Normally, these cells are quickly sequestered by the spleen. Always after splenectomy, rarely also in hemolytic conditions and megaloblastic anemia, they are observed in erythrocytes at a rate of > 1‰.

These Howell-Jolly bodies are visible after normal panoptic staining. Supravital staining (see reticulocyte count, p. 11) may produce a few globular precipitates at the cell membrane, known as Heinz bodies. They are a rare phenomenon and may indicate the presence of unstable hemoglobins in rare familial or severe toxic hemolytic conditions (p. 144).

An ellipsoid, eosinophil-violet stained, delicately structured ring in erythrocytes is called a Cabot ring (Fig. **55 d**). It probably consists not, as its form might suggest, of remnants of the nuclear membrane, but of fibers from the mitotic spindle. Because these ring structures are sporadically seen in all severe anemias, no specific conclusions can be drawn from their presence, but in the absence of any other rationale for severe anemia they are compatible with the suspicion of an incipient idiopathic erythropoietic disorder (e.g., panmyelopathy or smoldering leukosis or leukemia).

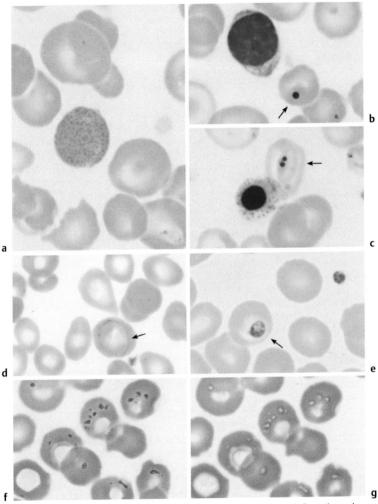

Fig. 55 Erythrocyte inclusions. **a** Polychromatic erythrocyte with fine, dense basophilic stippling. **b** Erythrocyte with Howell–Jolly bodies (arrow) in addition to a lymphocyte (after splenectomy). **c** Erythrocyte with two Howell–Jolly bodies (arrow) alongside an orthochromatic erythroblast with basophilic stippling (thalassemia, in this case with functional asplenia). **d** Erythrocyte with a delicate Cabot ring (arrow) (here in a case of osteomyelosclerosis). **e** Thrombocyte layered onto an erythrocyte (arrow). **f** and **g** Fixation and staining artifacts.

157

Hematological Diagnosis of Malaria

Various parasites may be found in the blood stream, e.g., trypanosomes and filariae. Among the parasitic diseases, probably only malaria is of practical diagnostic relevance in the northern hemisphere, while at the same time malarial involvement of erythrocytes may confuse the interpretation of erythrocyte morphology. For these reasons, a knowledge of the principal different morphological forms of malarial plasmodia is advisable.

Recurrent fever and influenza-like symptoms after a stay in tropical regions suggest malaria. The diagnosis may be confirmed from normal blood smears or thick smears; in the latter the erythrocytes have been hemolyzed and the pathogens exposed. Depending on the stage in the life cycle of the plasmodia, a variety of morphologically completely different forms may be found in the erythrocytes, sometimes even next to each other. The different types of pathogens show subtle specific differences that, once the referring physician suspects malaria, are best left to the specialist in tropical medicine, who will determine which of the following is the causative organism: *Plasmodium vivax* (tertian malaria), *Plasmodium falciparum* (falciparum or malignant tertian malaria) and *Plasmodium malariae* (quartan malaria) (Table **27**, Fig. **56**). Most cases of malaria are caused by *P. vivax* (42%) and *P. falciparum* (43%).

The key morphological characteristics in all forms of malaria can be summarized as the following basic forms: The first developmental stage of the pathogen, generally found in quite large erythrocytes, appears as small ring-shaped bodies with a central vacuole, called *trophozoites* (or the *signet-ring* stage) (Fig. **57**). The point-like center is usually most noticeable, as it is reminiscent of a Howell–Jolly body, and only a very careful search for the delicate ring form will supply the diagnosis. Occasionally, there are several signet-ring entities in one erythrocyte. All invaded cells may show reddish stippling, known as malarial stippling or Schüffner's dots. The pathogens keep dividing, progressively filling the vacuoles, and then develop into schizonts (Fig. **56**), which soon fill the entire erythrocyte with an average of 10–15 nuclei. Some schizonts have brown-black pigment inclusions. Finally the schizonts disintegrate, the erythrocyte ruptures, and the host runs a fever. The separate parts (*merozoites*) then start a new invasion of erythrocytes.

In parallel with asexual reproduction, merozoites develop into *gamonts*, which always remain mononuclear and can completely fill the erythrocyte with their stippled cell bodies. The large, dark blue-stained forms (macrogametes) are female cells (Fig. **57d**), the smaller, light blue-stained forms (microgametes) are male cells. Macrogametes usually predominate. They continue their development in the stomach of the infected *Anopheles* mosquito.

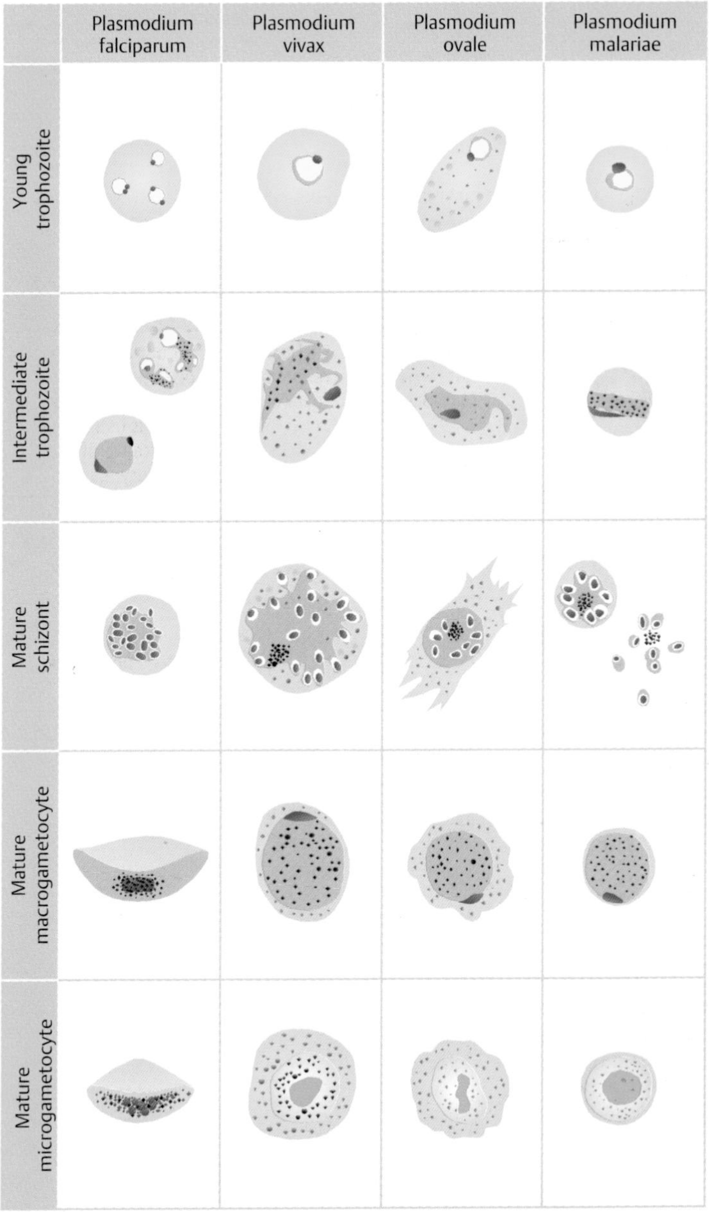

Fig. **56** Differential diagnosis of malaria plasmodia in a blood smear (from Kayser, F., et al., Medizinische Mikrobiologie (Medical Microbiology), Thieme, Stuttgart, 1993).

The example shown here is of the erythrocytic phases of *P. vivax*, because tertian malaria is the most common form of malaria and best shows the basic morphological characteristics of a plasmodia infection.

Table **27**   Parasitology of malaria and clinical characteristics (from Diesfeld, H., G. Krause: Praktische Tropenmedizin und Reisemedizin. Thieme, Stuttgart 1997)

Disease	Pathogen	Exoerythro-cytic phase ≅ incubation	Erythrocytic phase	Clinical charac-teristics
Falci-parum malaria	*Plasmodium falciparum*	7–15 days, does not form liver hypnozoites	48 hours, recurring fever is rare	Potentially lethal disease, widely therapy-resistant, there is usually no recurrence after recovery
Tertian malaria	*P. vivax*	12-18 days, forms liver hypnozoites	48 hours	Benign form recurrences up to 2 years after infection
	P. ovale			Benign form recurrences up to 5 years after infection
Quartan malaria	*P. malariae*	18-40 days, does not form liver hypnozoites	72 hours	Benign form recurrences possible up to 30 years after infection

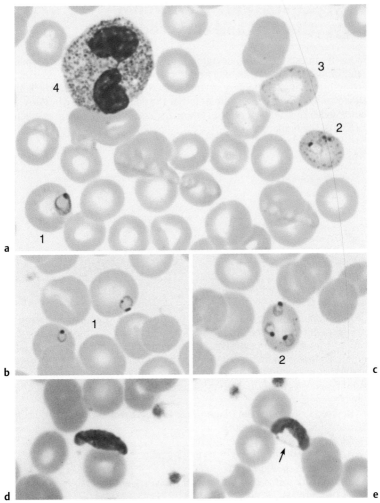

Fig. **57** Blood analysis in malaria. **a** Trophozoites in *Plasmodium falciparum* (falciparum or malignant tertian malaria) infection. Simple signet-ring form (1), double-invaded erythrocyte with basophilic stippling (2). Erythrocyte with basophilic stippling without plasmodium (3) and segmented neutrophilic granulocyte with toxic granulation (4). **b** and **c** *Plasmodium falciparum*: single invasion with delicate trophozoites (1), multiple invasion (2). **d** and **e** In the gametocyte stage of falciform malaria, the pathogens appear to reside outside the erythrocyte, but remnants of the erythrocyte membrane may be seen (arrow, **e**). For a systematic overview of malarial inclusions, see p. 159.

Polycythemia Vera (Erythremic Polycythemia) and Erythrocytosis

Increases in erythrocytes, hemoglobin, and hematocrit above the normal range *due to causes unrelated to hematopoiesis* (i.e., the majority of cases) are referred to as *secondary erythrocytosis* or *secondary polycythemia*. However, it should be remembered that the "normal" range of values is quite wide, especially for men, in whom the normal range can be as much as 55% of the hematocrit!

Table **28**   Causes of secondary erythrocytosis

Reduced O₂ transport capacity	– Carboxyhemoglobin formation in chronic smokers
	– High altitude hypoxia, COPD
	– Heart defect (right–left shunt)
	– Hypoventilation (e. g., obesity hypoventilation)
Reduced O₂ release from hemoglobin	– Congenital 2,3-diphosphoglycerate deficiency
Renal hypoxia	– Hydronephrosis, renal cyst
	– Renal artery stenosis
Autonomous erythropoietin biosynthesis	– Renal carcinoma
	– Adenoma

COPD = Chronic obstructive pulmonary disease

An *autonomous* increase in erythropoiesis, i.e., polycythemia vera, represents a very different situation. Polycythemia vera—which one might call a "primary erythrocytosis"—is a malignant stem cell abnormality of unknown origin and is a myeloproliferative syndrome (p. 112). Leukocyte counts (with increased basophils) and thrombocyte counts often rise simultaneously, and a transition to osteomyelosclerosis often occurs in the later stages.

Revised Criteria for the Diagnosis of Polycythemia Vera (according to Pearson and Messinezy, 1996)

— A1 elevated erythrocyte numbers
— A2 absence of any trigger of secondary polycythemia
— A3 palpable splenomegaly
— A4 clonality test, e.g., PRV-1 marker (polycythemia rubra vera 1)
— B1 thrombocytosis ($> 400 \times 10^9/l$)
— B2 leukocytosis ($> 10 \times 10^9/l$)
— B3 splenomegaly (sonogram)
— B4 endogenous erythrocytic colonies

Diagnosis in the presence of: A1 + A2 + A3/A4 or A1 + A2 + 2 × B

Bone marrow cytology shows increased erythropoiesis in both polycythemia vera and secondary polycythemia. Polycythemia vera is the more likely diagnosis when megakaryocytes, granulopoiesis, basophils, and eosinophils are also increased.

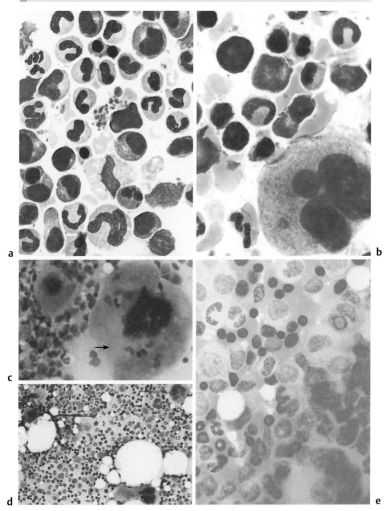

Fig. **58** Polycythemia vera and secondary erythrocytosis. **a** In reactive secondary erythrocytosis there is usually only an increase in erythropoiesis. **b** In polycythemia vera megakaryopoiesis (and often granulopoiesis) are also increased. **c** Bone marrow smear at low magnification in polycythemia vera, with a hyperlobulated megakaryocyte (arrow). **d** Bone marrow smear at low magnification in polycythemia vera, showing increased cell density and proliferation of megakaryocytes. **e** In polycythemia vera, iron staining shows no iron storage particles.

Thrombocyte Abnormalities

> ❗ EDTA in blood collection tubes (e.g., lavender top tubes) can lead to aggregation (pseudothrombocytopenia). A control using citrate as anti-coagulant is required.

The clinical sign of spontaneous bleeding in small areas of the skin and mucous membranes (petechial bleeding), which on injury diffuses out to form medium-sized subcutaneous ecchymoses, is grounds for suspicion of thrombocyte (or vascular) anomalies.

Thrombocytopenia

Thrombocytopenias Due to Increased Demand (High Turnover)

A characteristic sign of this pathology can be that among the few thrombocytes seen in the blood smear, there is an increased presence of larger, i.e., less mature cell forms.

The *bone marrow* in these thrombocytopenias shows raised (or at least normal) megakaryocyte counts. Here too, there may be an increased presence of less mature forms with one or two nuclei (Figs. **60, 61**).

Drug-induced immunothrombocytopenia As in drug-induced agranulocytosis, the process starts with an antibody response to a drug, or its metabolites, and binding of the antibody complex to thrombocytes. Rapid thrombocyte degradation by macrophages follows (Table **29**). The most common triggers are analgesic/anti-inflammatory drugs and antibiotics.

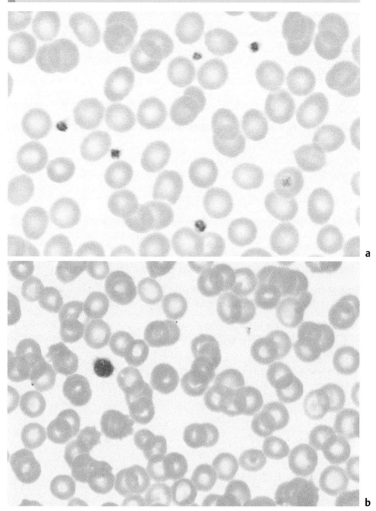

Fig. **59** Forms of thrombocytopenia. **a** This blood smear shows normal size and density of thrombocytes. **b** In this blood smear thrombocyte density is lower and size has increased, a feature typical of immunothrombocytopenia. *continued* ▶

Table **29** Most common triggers of drug-induced immunothrombocytopenia

Analgesics	Quinine	Isoniazid
Antibiotics	Digitalis preparations	Methyldopa
Anticonvulsive drugs	Furosemide	Spironolactone
Arsenic, e. g., in water	Gold salts	Tolbutamide
Quinidine	Heparin!	

"Idiopathic" immunothrombocytopenia. The name is largely historical, because often a trigger is found.

➤ Postinfectious = acute form, usually occurs in children after rubella, mumps, or measles.
➤ Essential thrombocytopenia, thrombocytopenic purpura (Werlhof disease)

Thrombocyte antibodies develop without an identifiable trigger. This is thus a primary autoimmune disease specifically targeting thrombocytes.

Secondary immunothrombocytopenias, e.g., in lupus erythematosus and other forms of immune vasculitis, lymphomas, and tuberculosis.

Post-transfusion purpura occurs mostly in women about one week after a blood transfusion, often after earlier transfusions or pregnancy.

Thrombocytopenia in microangiopathy. This group includes thrombotic–thrombocytopenic purpura (see p. 144) and disseminated intravascular coagulation.

Thrombocytopenia in hypersplenism of whatever etiology.

Fig. **59** Continued. **c** Pseudothrombocytopenia. The thrombocytes are not lying ▶ free and scattered around, but agglutinated together, leading to a reading of thrombocytopenia from the automated blood analyzer. **d** Giant thrombocyte (as large as an erythrocyte) in thrombocytopenia. Döhle-type bluish inclusion (arrow) in the normally granulated segmented neutrophilic granulocyte: May-Hegglin anomaly.

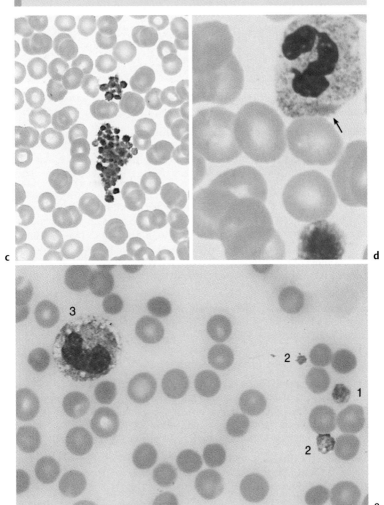

Fig. **59**   **e** Large thrombocyte (1) in thrombocytopenia. Thrombocyte-like fragments from destroyed granulocytes (cytoplasmic fragments) (2), which have the same structure and staining characteristics as the cytoplasm of band granulocytes (3). Clinical status of sepsis with disseminated intravascular coagulation. In automated counters cytoplasmic fragments are included in the thrombocyte fraction.

Thrombocytopenias Due to Reduced Cell Production

In this condition, blood contains few, usually small, pyknotic ("old") thrombocytes. Only a very few megakaryocytes are found in the bone marrow, and these have a normal appearance.

Causes

Chronic alcoholism. There may be some overlap with increased turnover and folic acid deficiency.

Chemical and radiological noxae. Cytostatics naturally lead directly to a dose-dependent reduction in megakaryocyte counts. A large therapeutic radiation burden in the area of blood-producing bone marrow has the same result, which may persist for many months.

Virus infections. Measles, mononucleosis (Epstein–Barr virus, cytomegalovirus), rubella, and influenza may (usually in children) trigger thrombocytopenias of various types. In these cases, the virus affects the megakaryocytes directly. However, antibodies to thrombocytes may also arise in the course of these infections (p. 166), so that the pathomechanism of the parainfectious thrombocytopenias described by Werlhof in children may lie in impaired production and/or increased degradation of thrombocytes.

Neoplastic and aplastic bone marrow diseases. All neoplasms of the bone marrow cell series (e.g., leukemia, lymphoma, and plasmacytoma), together with their precursor forms (e.g., myelodysplasia), lead to progressive thrombocytopenia, as do panmyelophthisis and bone marrow infiltration by metastases from solid tumors.

Vitamin deficiency. Folic acid and vitamin B_{12} deficiencies from various causes (p. 152) also affect the rapidly proliferating megakaryocytes. In these cases, thrombocytopenia is often present before anemia and leukocytopenia in circulating blood, while the bone marrow shows copious megakaryocytes that have been blocked from maturation.

Constitutional diseases. An amegakaryocytic thrombocytopenia without any of the above causes is rare. It is seen in children with congenital radial aplasia; in adults it tends usually to be an early sign of leukemia, myelodysplastic syndrome, or aplastic anemia.

Wiscott-Aldrich syndrome (thrombocytopenia, immune deficiency, and eczema) is an X-chromosomal recessive disease in boys and presents with thrombocytopenia with ineffective megakaryopoiesis.

The *May-Hegglin anomaly* (dominant hereditary transmission) is characterized by thrombocytopenia with giant thrombocytes and granulocyte inclusions, which resemble Döhle bodies (endoplasmatic reticulum aggregates).

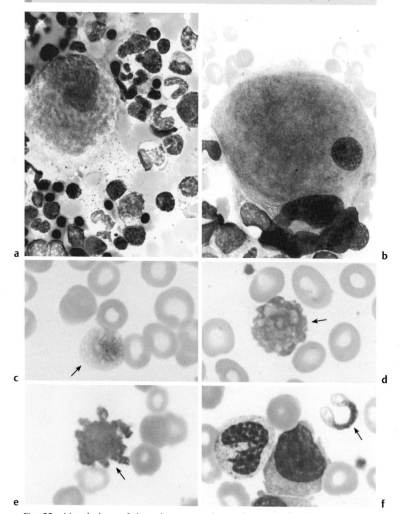

Fig. **60** Morphology of thrombocytes and megakaryocytes. **a** Bone marrow in
thrombocytopenia due to increased turnover (e.g., immunothrombocytopenia).
Mononuclear "young" megakaryocytes clearly budding a thrombocyte (irregular,
cloudy cytoplasm structure). **b** In thrombocytopenia against a background of
myelodysplasia, the bone marrow shows various megakaryocyte anomalies: here,
too small a nucleus surrounded by too wide cytoplasm. **c–f** In myelodysplasia
(**c** and **d**) and acute myeloid leukemia (**e** and **f**), bizarre anomalous thrombocyte
shapes (arrows) may occasionally be found.

169

Thrombocytosis (Including Essential Thrombocythemia)

Reactive. Thrombocytosis in the form of a constant *elevation* of thrombocyte counts above an upper normal range of 300 000–450 000/μl, may be *reactive*, i.e., may appear in response to various tumors (particularly bronchial carcinoma), chronic inflammation (particularly ulcerative colitis, primary chronic polyarthritis), bleeding, or iron deficiency. The pathology of this form is not known.

Essential Thrombocythemia

Essential thrombocythemia, by contrast, is a myeloproliferative disease (see p. 114) in which the main feature of increased thrombocytes is accompanied by other signs of this group of diseases that may vary in severity, such as leukocytosis and an enlarged spleen. Severe thrombocythemia may also be seen in osteomyelosclerosis, polycythemia vera, and chronic myeloid leukemia, and for this reason the following specific diagnostic criteria have been suggested:

   Diagnostic criteria for essential thrombocytopenia (according to Murphy et al.)

➤ Thrombocytes $> 600 \times 10^9$/l (with control)
➤ Normal erythrocyte mass or Hb < 18.5 g/dl ♂, 16.5 g/dl ♀
➤ No significant bone marrow fibrosis
➤ No splenomegaly
➤ No leukoerythroblastic CBC
➤ Absence of morphological or cytogenetic criteria of myelodysplasia
➤ Secondary thrombocytosis (iron deficiency, inflammation, neoplasia, trauma, etc.) excluded

Large thrombocytes are found in the *peripheral blood* smear. However, these also occur in polycythemia vera and osteomyelosclerosis.
   Bone marrow cytology will show markedly elevated megakaryocyte counts, with the cells often forming clusters and often with hypersegmented nuclei.

Fig. **61**   Essential thrombocythemia. **a** Increased thrombocyte density and marked anisocytosis in essential thrombocythemia. **b** Large thrombocytes (1) and a micro(mega)karyocyte nucleus (2) in essential thrombocythemia. Micro(mega)karyocytes are characterized by a small, very dense and often lobed nucleus with narrow, uneven cytoplasm, the processes of which correspond to thrombocytes (arrow). ▶

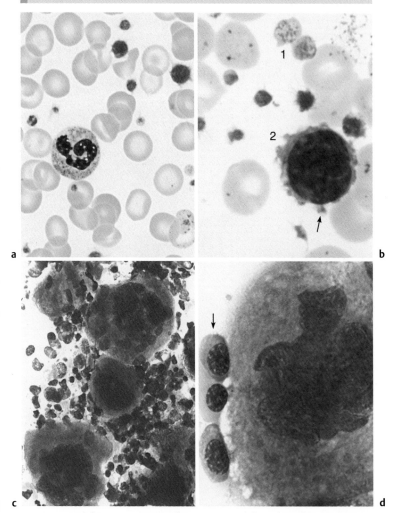

a

b

c

d

Fig. **61** **c** and **d** Bone marrow cytology in essential thrombocythemia: there is a striking abundance of very large, hyperlobulated megakaryocytes (**c**); such megakaryocytes may also be seen in polycythemia vera. **d** Size comparison with basophilic erythroblasts (arrow). The cloudy cytoplasm of the megakaryocyte is typical of effective thrombocyte production.

171

Cytology of Organ Biopsies and Exudates*

* Special thanks to Dr. T. Binder, Wuppertal, for the generous gift of several preparations.

In this guide to morphology, only a basic indication can be given of the materials that may be drawn upon for a cytological diagnosis and what basic kinds of information cytology is able to give.

For specialized cytological organ diagnostics, the reader should refer to a suitable cytology atlas. Often appropriately prepared samples are often sent away to a hematological–cytological or a pathoanatomic laboratory for analysis. Thus, the images in this chapter are intended particularly to help the clinician understand the interpretation of samples that he or she has not investigated in person.

In principle, *all parenchymatous organs* can be accessed for material for cytological analysis. Of particular importance are thyroid biopsy (especially in the region of scintigraphically "cold" nodules), liver and spleen biopsy (under laparascopic guidance) in the region of lumps lying close to the surface, and breast and prostate biopsy. Again, the cytological analysis is usually made by a specialist cytologist or pathologist.

Lymph node cytology, effusion cytology (pleura, ascites), cerebrospinal fluid cytology, and bronchial lavage are usually the responsibility of the internist with a special interest in morphology and are closely related to hemato-oncology.

Lymph Node Cytology

The *diagnosis of enlarged lymph nodes* receives special attention here because lymph nodes are as important as bone marrow for hematopoiesis. While in most instances abnormalities in the bone marrow cell series can be detected from the peripheral blood, this is very rarely the case for lymphomas. For this reason, lymph node cytology, a relatively simple and well-tolerated technique (p. 24), is critically important for the guidance it can give about the cause of enlarged lymph nodes. Figure **62** offers a diagnostic flow chart.

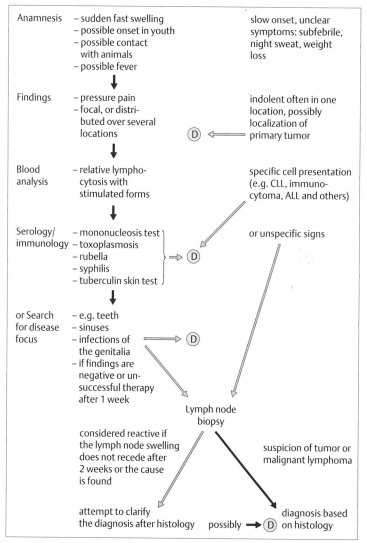

Fig. **62** Diagnostic flow chart for cases of lymph node enlargement. (D) Diagnosis.

Reactive Lymph Node Hyperplasia and Lymphogranulomatosis (Hodgkin Disease)

Reactive lymph node hyperplasia of whatever etiology is characterized by a confused mixture of small, middle-sized, and large lymphocytes. When the latter have a nuclear diameter at least three times the size of the predominating small lymphocytes and have a fair width of basophilic cytoplasm, they are called immunoblasts (lymphoblasts). Cells with deeply basophilic, eccentric cytoplasm and dense nuclei are called plasmablasts, and cells with a narrow cytoplasmic seam are centroblasts. Lymphocytes can also to varying degrees show a tendency to appear as plasma cells, e.g., as plasmacytoid lymphocytes with a relatively wide seam of cytoplasm. Monocytes and phagocytic macrophages are also seen (Fig. **63**).

Table **30** (p. 178) summarizes the different forms of reactive lymphadenitis. The basic cytological findings in all of them is always a complete mixture of small to very large lymphocytes. Occasionally more specific findings may indicate the possibility of mononucleosis (increased immature monocytes) or toxoplasmosis (plasmablasts, phagocytic macrophages, and possibly epithelioid cells).

> **ℹ** Any enlargement of the lymph nodes that persists for more than two weeks should be subjected to histological analysis unless the history, clinical findings, serology, or CBC offer an explanation.

At first sight, the confusion visible in the cytological findings of *lymphogranulomatosis (Hodgkin disease)* is reminiscent of the picture in reactive hyperplasia (something which may be important for an understanding of the pathology of this disease compared with other malignant neoplasms). However, some cells elements show signs of a strong immunological "over-reaction" in which large, immunoblast-like cells form with well-developed nucleoli (Hodgkin cells). Sporadically, some of these cells are found to be multinucleated (Reed–Sternberg giant cells); infiltrations of eosinophils and plasma cells may also be found. Findings of this type always require histological analysis, which can distinguish between four prognostically relevant histological subtypes. In addition to this, the very lack of a clear demarcation between Hodgkin disease and reactive conditions is reason enough to conduct a histological study of every lymph node that appears reactive if does not regress completely within two weeks.

In cases of histologically verified Hodgkin disease, cytological analysis is especially useful in the assessment of new lymphomas after therapy.

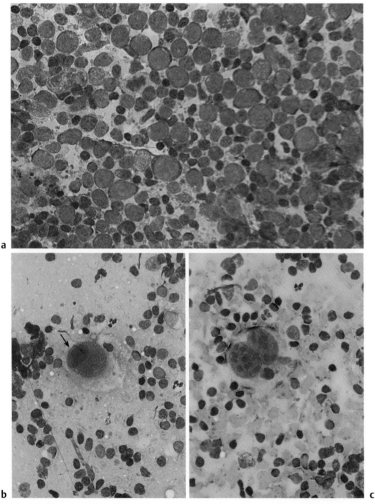

Fig. **63** Reactive lymph node hyperplasia and lymphogranulomatosis. **a** Lymph node cytology in severe reactive hyperplasia. Large blastic cells alongside small lymphocytes (if it fails to regress, histological analysis is required). **b** Hodgkin disease: a giant mononuclear cell with a large nucleolus (arrow) and wide cytoplasmic layer (Hodgkin cell), surrounded by small and medium-sized lymphocytes. **c** Hodgkin disease: giant binuclear cell (Reed–Sternberg giant cell).

Table 30 Sequence of steps in the diagnosis of reactive lymphoma

Anamnesis	Symptoms	Tentative diagnosis	Diagnostic studies	Cytology	Histology
Rapid progression (fever)	Localized, painful	**Perifocal lymphadenitis**	Search for disease focus, non-specific changes in CBC and ESR	(→) Non-specific lymphadenitis	
Rapid progression, fever, sore throat	Diffuse, painfull; angina, possibly spleen	**Mononucleosis**	Pfeiffer cells in the blood analysis, EBV serology (1)	(→) Adenitis with histiocytosis	
Most children	Nuchal lymph nodes, later exanthema	**Rubella**	Plasma cells in the blood, rubella-AHT ↑ (2)		
Ingestion of raw meat Contact with cats	Diffuse	**Toxoplasmosis**	Serology (3)	(→) With epithelioid cells and macrophages	Epithelioid cell lymphadenitis
Pharyngitis (+ conjunctivitis)	Local Neck area	**Common viruses, specific adenoviruses**	Complement fixation reaction (adenoviruses, less commonly coxsackieviruses) (4)		
Slow growth, general malaise	Inflamed lymph nodes, possibly fistulae	**Tuberculosis**	Thorax, local primary infections, skin test, pathogen in biopsy aspirate, possibly PCR	(→) Epithelioid cells, Langhans giant cells	
Slow growth	Hard; possibly skin infiltrations	**Sarcoidosis (Boeck disease)**	Thorax, tuberculin test usually negative, ACE	→ Epithelioid cells	Epithelioid cell fibrosis

Contact with animals	Tonsillitis, neck lymph nodes	**Listeriosis**	Agglutination test, complement fixation reaction	(→) It may be possible to determine the pathogen from the biopsy
Contact with animals Milk intake	Fever, spleen	**Brucellosis**	In case of fever: pathogen in blood, serology	
Open wound, possibly from a cat	Local primary lesion	**Cat-scratch disease**	Leukocytosis, lymphocytosis, complement fixation reaction	→ Epithelioid cells, giant cells — Perforating lymphadenitis
Contact with wildlife	Local primary lesion	**Tularemia (rabbit fever)**	Agglutination test	
Little sense of illness	Inflamed hard infiltrates, possibly fistulae	**Actinomycosis**	Leukocytosis, left shift	→ "Gland" tissue in the biopsy material — Therapeutic excision
Symptomatic joints	Joints, spleen, possibly kidney	**Collagen disease (PCP, LE) Felty syndrome, Still disease**	Antinuclear factor	
No symptoms	Submandibular swelling, no irritation	**Branchial cyst**		→ Epithelial cells, macrophages, and granulocytes — Therapeutic excision

(→) = Optional step; → = usually diagnostic step, if there is no arrow, the diagnosis can be made on the basis of preceding steps. (1) = Positive from day 5; (2) = 1–4 days after exanthema, may be as much as 1 month; (3) = from week 4; (4) = from day 10.

Sarcoidosis and Tuberculosis

The material of cell biopsies taken from indolent, nonirritated enlarged lymph nodes in the neck or axilla that have developed with little in the way of clinical symptoms, or from subcutaneous infiltration in various regions, can be quite homogeneous. With their thin, very long, ovoid nucleus (four to five times the size of lymphocytes), delicate reticular chromatin structure, and extensive layer of cytoplasm that may occasionally appear confluent with that of other cells, they are reminiscent of the epithelial cells that line the body's internal cavities and are therefore called epithelioid cells. They are known to be the tissue form of transformed monocytes, and are found in increased numbers in *all chronic inflammatory processes*—especially toxoplasmosis, autoimmune diseases, and foreign-body reactions—and also in the neighborhood and drainage areas of tumors. They exclusively dominate the cytological picture in a particular form of chronic "inflammation," *sarcoidosis* (*Boeck disease*). A typical finding almost always encountered at the pulmonary hilus combined with a negative tuberculin test will all but confirm this diagnosis. The appearance of a few multinuclear cells (Langhans giant cells) may allow confusion with tuberculosis, but clinical findings and a tuberculin skin test will usually make the diagnosis clear.

Rapidly developing, usually hard, pressure-sensitive neck lymph nodes, seemingly connected with each other with some fluctuant zones and external inflammatory redness, suggest the now rare scrofulous form of *tuberculosis*. A highly positive tuberculin skin test also suggests this diagnosis. If any remaining doubts cannot be dispelled clinically, a very-fine-needle lymph node biopsy may be performed, but only if the skin shows noninflammatory, pale discoloration.

The harvested material can show the potency of the tissue-bound forms of cells in the monocyte/macrophage series. In addition to mononuclear epithelioid cells, there are giant cell conglomerates made up of polynuclear epithelioid cells in enormous syncytia with 10, 20, or more nuclei. These are called *Langhans giant cells*. In scrofuloderma (tuberculosis colliquativa), there are also lymphocytic and granulocytic cells in the process of degradation, which are absent in purely productive tuberculous lymphadenitis.

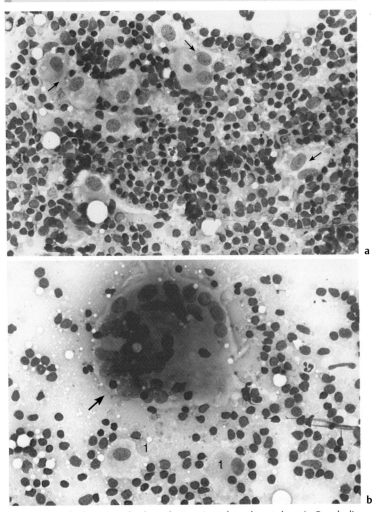

Fig. **64** Boeck disease and tuberculosis. **a** Lymph node cytology in Boeck disease: a special form of reactive cell pattern with (often predominating) islands and trains of epithelioid cells (arrow), which have ovoid nuclei with delicate chromatin structure and a wide, smoke-gray layer of cytoplasm. **b** Lymph node cytology in tuberculous lymphadenitis: in addition to lymphocytes and a few epithelial cells (1), enormous syncytes of epithelioid cell nuclei within one cytoplasm (arrow) may be encountered: the Langhans giant cell.

181

Non-Hodgkin Lymphoma

Since the CBC is the first step in any lymph node diagnosis, lymph node biopsy is unnecessary in many cases of non-Hodgkin lymphoma (p. 70), because the most common form of this group of diseases, chronic lymphadenosis, can always be diagnosed on the basis of the leukemic findings of the CBC.

However, when enlarged lymph nodes are found in one or more regions without symptoms of reactive disease, and the blood analysis fails to show signs of leukemia, lymph node biopsy is indicated.

> The relatively monotonous lymph node cytology in non-Hodgkin lymphomas and tumor metastases mean that histological differentiation is required.

In contrast to Hodgkin disease, with its conspicuous giant cell forms (p. 177), non-Hodgkin lymphomas display a monotonous picture without any signs of a reactive process (p. 70). Clinically, it is enough to distinguish between small cell forms (which have a relatively good prognosis) and large cell forms (which have a poorer prognosis) to begin with. For a more detailed classification, see page 70 f.

Histological analysis may be omitted only when its final results would not be expected to add to the intermediate cytological findings in terms of consequences for treatment.

Metastases of Solid Tumors in Lymph Nodes or Subcutaneous Tissue

When hard nodules are found that are circumscribed in location, biopsy shows aggregates of polymorphous cells with mostly undifferentiated nuclei and a coarse reticular structure of the chromatin (perhaps with well-defined nucleoli or nuclear vacuoles), and the lymphatic cells cannot be classified, there is urgent suspicion of metastasis from a *malignant solid tumor,* i.e. from a carcinoma in a variety of possible locations or a soft tissue sarcoma.

> As a rule, the next step is the search for a possible primary tumor. If this is found, lymph node resection becomes unnecessary.

If no primary tumor is found, lymph node histology is indicated. The histological findings can provide certain clues about the etiology and also helps in the difficult differential diagnosis versus blastic non-Hodgkin lymphoma.

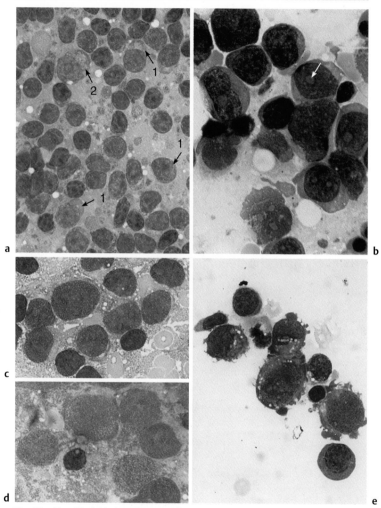

Fig. **65** Non-Hodgkin lymphoma and tumor metastases. **a** Lymph node cytology showing small cells with relatively wide cytoplasm (arrow 1) in addition to lymphocytes. There are scattered blasts with wide cytoplasm (arrow 2): lymphoplasmacytic immunocytoma. **b** Lymph node cytology showing exclusively large blastoid cells with a large central nucleolus (arrow). This usually indicates large-cell non-Hodgkin lymphoma (in this case immunoblastic). **c–e** Metastatic disease from: **c** uterine carcinoma, **d** small-cell bronchial carcinoma, and **e** leiomyosarcoma.

183

Branchial Cysts and Bronchoalveolar Lavage

Branchial Cysts

A (usually unilateral) swollen neck nodule below the mandibular angle that feels firm to pressure, but is without external signs of inflammation, should suggest the presence of a branchial cyst. Surprisingly, aspiration usually produces a brownish-yellow liquid. In addition to partially cytolysed granulocytes and lymphocytes (cell detritus), a smear of this liquid, or the centrifuged precipitate, shows cells with small central nuclei and wide light cell centers which are identical to epithelial cells from the floor of the mouth. Biopsies from a soft swelling around the larynx show the same picture; in this case it is a retention cyst from another developmental remnant, the *ductus thyroglossus.*

Cytology of the Respiratory System, Especially Bronchoalveolar Lavage

Through the development of patient-friendly endoscopic techniques, diagnostic lavage (with 10–30 ml physiological saline solution) and its cytological workup are now in widespread use. This method is briefly mentioned here because of its broad interest for all medical professionals with an interest in morphology; the interested reader is referred to the specialist literature (e.g. Costabel, 1994) for further information. Table **31** lists the most important indications for bronchoalveolar lavage.

Table **31**   Clinical indications for bronchoalveolar lavage (according to Costabel 1994)

Interstitial infiltrates	Alveolar infiltrates	Pulmonary infiltrates in patients with immune deficiency
Sarcoidosis (Boeck disease)	Pneumonia	HIV Infection
Exogenous allergic alveolitis	Alveolar hemorrhage	Treatment with cytostatic agents
Drug-induced alveolitis	Alveolar proteinosis	Radiation sickness
Idiopathic pulmonary fibrosis	Eosinophilic pneumonia	Immunosuppressive therapy
Collagen disease	Obliterating bronchiolitis	Organ transplant
Histiocytosis X		
Pneumoconioses		
Lymphangiosis carcinomatosa		

Accessible cysts (e.g., branchial cysts) should be aspirated. Bronchial lavage is a cytological new discipline

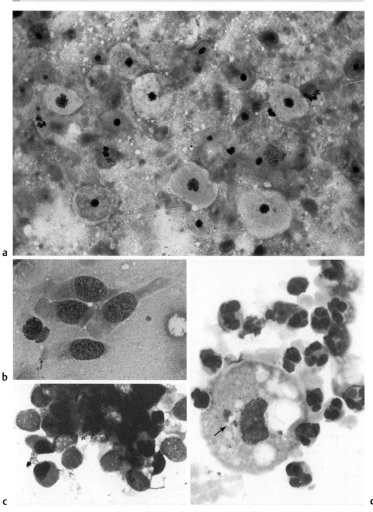

Fig. **66** Cyst biopsy and bronchoalveolar lavage. **a** Cytology of a lateral neck cyst: no lymphatic tissue, but epithelial cells from the floor of the mouth. **b** Normal ciliated epithelial cells with typical cytoplasmic processes. **c** Tumor cell conglomeration in small-cell bronchial carcinoma: conglomeration is typical of tumor cells. **d** Bronchoalveolar lavage in purulent bronchitis: a macrophage with pigment inclusion (arrow) is surrounded by segmented neutrophilic granulocytes.

185

Cytology of Pleural Effusions and Ascites

> Pleural effusions always require cytological diagnostic procedures unless they are secondary to a known disease, such as cardiac insufficiency or pneumonia, and recede on treatment of the primary disease.

Pleura aspirates can be classified as exudates or transudates (the latter usually caused by hydrodynamic stasis). The specific density (measured with a simple areometer) of transudates, which are protein-poor, is between 1008 and 1015 g/l, while for exudates it is greater than 1018 g/l.

Cytological preparation may be done by gentle centrifugation of the aspirate (10 minutes at 300–500 rpm), which should be as fresh as possible; the supernatant is decanted and the sediment suspended in the residual fluid, which will collect on the bottom of the centrifuge tube. Nowadays, however, this procedure has been replaced by cytocentrifugation.

Effusions that are noticeably rich in eosinophilic granulocytes should raise the suspicion of Hodgkin disease, generalized reaction to the presence of a tumor, or an allergic or autoimmune disorder. Purely lymphatic effusions are particularly suggestive of tuberculosis. In addition, all transudates and exudates contain various numbers of endothelial cells (particularly high in cases of bacterial pleuritis) that have been sloughed off from the pleural lining.

Any cell elements that do not fulfill the above criteria should be regarded as suspect for neoplastic transformation, especially if they occur in aggregates. Characteristics that in general terms support such a suspicion include extended size polymorphy, coarse chromatin structure, well-defined nucleoli, occasional polynucleated cells, nuclear and plasma vacuoles, and deep cytoplasmic basophilia. For practical reasons, special diagnostic procedures should always be initiated in these situations.

What was said above in relation to the cell composition of pleural effusions also holds for ascites. Here too, the specific density may be determined and the Rivalta test to distinguish exudate from transudate carried out. Inflammatory exudates usually have a higher cell content; a strong predominance of lymphocytes may indicate tuberculosis. Like the pleura, the peritoneum is lined by phagocytotic endothelial cells which slough off into the ascitic fluid and, depending on the extent of the fluid, may produce a polymorphous overall picture analogous to that of the pleural endothelial cells. It is not always easy to distinguish between such endothelial cells and malignant tumor metastases. However, the latter usually occur not alone but in coherent cell aggregates ("floating metastases"), the various individual elements of which typically show a coarse chromatin structure, wide variation in size, well-defined nucleoli, and deeply basophilic cytoplasm.

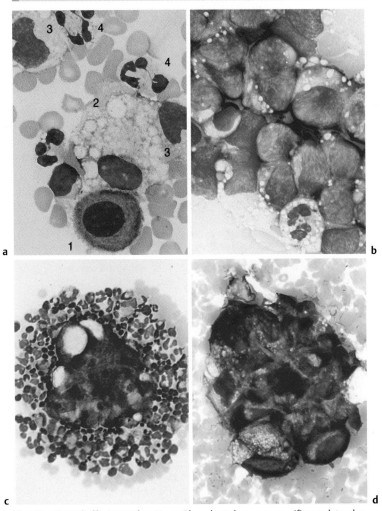

Fig. **67** Pleural effusion and ascites. **a** Pleural cytology, nonspecific exudate: dormant mesothelial cell (or serosal cover cell) (1), phagocytic macrophage with vacuoles (2), and monocytes (3), in addition to segmented neutrophilic granulocytes (4). **b** Cell composition in a pleural aspirate (prepared using a cytocentrifuge): variable cells, whose similarity to cells in acute leukemia should be established by cytochemistry and marker analysis: lymphoblastic lymphoma. **c** Ascites with tumor cell conglomerate, surrounded with granulocytes and monocytes, in this case of ovarian carcinoma. **d** Ascites cytology with an island of tumor cells. This kind of conglomeration is typical of tumor cells.

187

Cytology of Cerebrospinal Fluid

The first step in all hemato-oncological and neurological diagnostic assessments of cerebrospinal fluid is the quantitative and *qualitative* analysis of the cell composition (Table **32**).

Table **32** Emergency diagnostics of the liquor (according to Felgenhauer in Thomas 1998)

> ➤ Pandy's reaction
> ➤ Cell count (Fuchs-Rosenthal chamber)
> ➤ Smear (or cytocentrifuge preparation)
>   – to analyze the cell differentiation and
>   – to search for bacteria and roughly determine their types and prevalence
> ➤ Gram stain
> ➤ An additional determination of bacterial antigens may be done

Using advanced cell diagnostic methods, lymphocyte subpopulations can be identified by immunocytology and marker analysis and cytogenetic tests carried out on tumor cells.

Prevalence of neutrophilic granulocytes with strong pleocytosis suggests bacterial meningitis; often the bacteria can be directly characterized.

Prevalence of lymphatic cells with moderate pleocytosis suggests viral meningitis. (If clinical and serological findings leave doubts, the differential diagnosis must rule out lymphoma using immunocytological methods.)

Strong eosinophilia suggests parasite infection (e.g., cysticercosis).

A complete mixture of cells with granulocytes, lymphocytes, and monocytes in equal proportion is found in tuberculous meningitis.

Variable blasts, usually with significant pleocytosis, predominate in leukemic or lymphomatous meningitis.

Undefinable cells with large nuclei suggest tumor cells in general, e.g., meningeal involvement in breast cancer or bronchial carcinoma, etc. The cell types are determined on the basis of knowledge of the primary tumor and/or by marker analysis. Among primary brain tumors, the most likely cells to be found in cerebrospinal fluid are those from ependymoma, pinealoma, and medulloblastoma.

Erythrophages and siderophages (siderophores) are monocytes/macrophages, which take up erythrocytes and iron-containing pigment during subarachnoid hemorrhage.

> **!** The cytological analysis of the cerebrospinal fluid offers important clues to the character of meningeal inflammation, the presence of a malignancy, or hemorrhage.

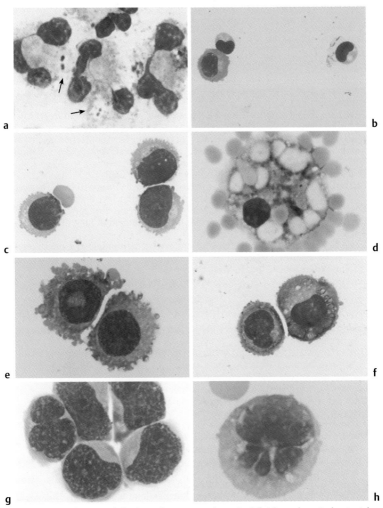

Fig. **68** Cerebrospinal fluid cytology. **a** Cerebrospinal fluid cytology in bacterial meningitis: granulocytes with phagocytosed diplococci (in this case, pneumococci, arrow). **b** Cerebrospinal fluid cytology in viral meningitis: variable lymphoid cells. **c** Cerebrospinal fluid cytology in non-Hodgkin lymphoma: here, mantle cell lymphoma. **d** Cerebrospinal fluid cytology after subarachnoid hemorrhage: macrophages with phagocytosed erythrocytes. **e–h** Cerebrospinal fluid cytology in meningeal involvement in malignancy: the origin of the cells cannot be deduced with certainty from the spinal fluid cytology alone: (**e**) breast cancer, (**f**) bronchial carcinoma, (**g**) medulloblastoma, and (**h**) acute leukemia. **189**

References

Begemann, H., M. Begemann: Praktische Hämatologie, 10. Aufl. Thieme, Stuttgart 1998

Begemann, H., J. Rastetter: Klinische Hämatologie, 4. Aufl. Thieme, Stuttgart 1993

Bessis, M.: Blood Smears Reinterpreted. Springer, Berlin 1977

Binet, J.L., A. Auquier, G. Dighiero et al.: A new prognostic classification of chronic lymphocytic leukemia derived from a multivariate survival analysis. Cancer 1981; 48(1): 198-206

Brücher, H.: Knochenmarkzytologie. Thieme, Stuttgart 1986

Classen, M., A. Dierkesmann, H. Heimpel et al.: Rationelle Diagnostik und Therapie in der inneren Medizin. Urben & Schwarzenberg, München 1996

Costabel, M.: Atlas der bronchoalveolären Lavage. Thieme, Stuttgart 1994

Costabel V., J. Guzman: Bronchoalveolar lavage in interstital lung disease. Curr Opin Pulm Med 2001; 7(5): 255-61

Durie, B.G.M., S.E. Salmon: A clinical staging system for multiple myeloma. Correlation of measured myeloma cell mass with presenting clinical features, response to treatment, and survival. Cancer 1975; 36: 842-854

Heckner, F., M. Freund: Praktikum der mikroskopischen Hämatologie. Urban & Schwarzenberg, München 1994

Heimpel, H., D. Hoelzer, E. Kleihauer, H. P. Lohrmann: Hämatologie in der Praxis. Fischer, Stuttgart 1996

Huber, H., H. Löffler, V. Faber: Methoden der diagnostischen Hämatologie. Springer, Berlin 1994

Jaffe, E. S., N. L. Harris, H. Stein, J. W. Vardiman: World Health Organization Classification of Tumours. Pathology and Genetics of Tumours of Haematopoietic and Lymphoid Tissues. IARC Press, Lyon 2001

Lennert, K., A. C. Feller: Non-Hodgkin-Lymphome. Springer, Berlin 1990

Löffler, H., J. Rastetter: Atlas der klinischen Hämatologie. Springer, Berlin 1999

Murphy, S.: Diagnostic criteria and prognosis in polycythemia vera and essential thombocythemia. Semin Hematol 1999; 36(1 Suppl 2): 9-13

Ovell, S. R., G. Sterrett, M. N. Walters, D. Whitaker: Fine Needle Aspiration Cytology. Churchill Livingstone, Edinburgh London 1992

Pearson, T.C., M Messinezy: The diagnostic criteria of polycythaemia rubra vera. Leuk Lymphoma 1996;22(Suppl 1): 87-93

Pralle, H. B.: Checkliste Hämatologie, 2. Aufl. Thieme, Stuttgart 1991

Schmoll, H. J., K. Höffken, K. Possinger: Kompendium internistische Onkologie, 3. Bde., 3. Aufl. Springer, Berlin 1999

Theml, H., W. Kaboth, H. Begemann: Blutkrankheiten. In Kühn, H. A., J. Schirmeister: Innere Medizin, 5. Aufl. Springer, Berlin 1989

Theml, H., H. D. Schick: Praktische Differentialdiagnostik hämatologischer und onkologischer Krankheiten. Thieme, Stuttgart 1998

Zucker-Franklin, D., M. F. Greaves, C. E. Grossi, A. M. Marmont: Atlas der Blutzellen, 2. Aufl. Fischer, Stuttgart 1990

Index